CW01501978

ACKNOWLEDGMENTS

Thanks to Gwyn, who was the first person to read the entire book cover to cover and who's copy editing improved it 10-fold making it infinitely more readable.

Thank you to my loving husband Cormac, or should I say my long-suffering husband, who right from the early days took up the slack with the baby-minding to allow me to train. Many men wouldn't. He knew how much I needed to get out for my sanity, never mind my fitness.

My mum was a rock of support. Much as she doesn't understand my obsession with exercise and my drive to compete, without question she has always been behind me. From frequent trips to Dublin to mind Tori while I went out on my bike to minding her while I was at the worlds in Manchester, she helped make it all possible. And all the time Dad silently supported her in turn, supporting me.

Finally, thanks to my coach Hugh, who never sees limits, gets the best out of me and always finds a way through.

PREGNANCY TO PODIUM

Pregnancy to Podium
My journey challenging the myths about exercise with bump and beyond

Susie Mitchell

ISBN: 1492994693
ISBN-13: 978-1492994695

DEDICATION

To Tori, my beautiful daughter,
and to pregnant women everywhere, go for it!

PREGNANCY TO PODIUM

CONTENTS

PREGNANCY TO PODIUM

PROLOGUE

You can prepare, but nothing prepares you for it. The impact of having a baby on your life is colossal.

Would there ever be time for anything else? Would I ever have the energy for anything else? How would I cope when I had to travel up and down the country visiting fish farms, and was my new passion for track cycling over before it had begun?

For nine months she had gone everywhere with me, my little training partner. We had rolled miles in the countryside, participated in spinning classes, lifted weights, swam kilometres, but somehow now it was different. Who would have thought it would be a lot harder with her on the outside.

My goal had been to arrive at the birth of my baby in peak physical condition. It became my focus during pregnancy. I had achieved this and in ways was probably fitter then I ever had been. I had trained with my bump in ways I never thought possible, and had enjoyed every minute of it. It was a journey of discovery. Sometimes it was hard but I had found a way and felt on top of things as my due date rolled around.

However, when my beautiful healthy baby arrived into the world, everything went out the window. I had a dose of reality to deal with, grappling with the concept of being responsible for another human being for the rest of my life. I watched people through my window cycling past as I sat inside in my pyjamas trying to feed my baby and wondered would I ever get out and ride my bike again. I was physically exhausted from lack of sleep, frayed after surgery, but more importantly I was mentally falling apart. I started to wonder if I was ever going to feel normal or be as happy and carefree as before. The whole experience, to my utter shock, had totally floored me. Now I finally knew what people were talking about when they told me I had no idea what was ahead.

Two weeks later, I would make my first tentative steps back to fitness, and much more.

SUSIE MITCHELL

A JOURNEY BEGINS -
ADVENTURE RACING TO BABIES & BIKES

Before I write anything else, I want to explain why I decided to write this book. Right from the early days of my pregnancy, and even before, I became acutely aware of how little sound information was out there for women who wanted to continue exercising at a reasonable level while expecting. I couldn't understand it at first, but I realised pretty quickly what the problem was. No one wants to give pregnant women anything other than the most conservative advice just in case something happens to them while exercising. Much as I resented and was annoyed by that, I could understand it.

Since I couldn't find a book to read that gave me what I had searched for, I decided to try writing one myself. I thought I had a clear plan when I started out, but it turned out that I was way off the mark. From talking to several expectant mothers and from a survey I performed, I realised not only is every woman and her ability to tolerate exercise at varying intensities different, but every pregnancy is different, and every stage of pregnancy is, of course, also different. That's a lot of variables to have to deal with.

For a few weeks I thought of abandoning the idea, but this did not sit well with me. I realised as my pregnancy and early days with the baby went on I still wanted to write something, but wasn't sure of how to approach it. It was then I came up with the idea of a story. Instead of telling pregnant women what they should do, I'd tell them what I did, about my experiences and the knowledge I gathered through my research, and empower them to make up their own minds. I realised I had a story to tell, one very much defined by my own personal experiences both during and after the pregnancy.

There was more to my story than the type of exercise I did during the second trimester. Mine was a story about a woman whose personality had been defined by her passion for sport and competition and how she was afraid that pregnancy and becoming a mum might change all that. It was also about a woman getting to grips with coping with becoming a mum for the first time and the impact it had on her life. I knew for sure that in the early days when I was feeling a bit low and struggling to cope I would have loved more than anything to read about someone in a similar situation.

The unexpected happy ending to this tale was just the icing on the cake. I never could have imagined that carrying and having my beautiful baby Tori would lead to my fulfilling a lifelong dream of becoming a sporting champion.

I am a 37 year old woman and recreational athlete who thrives on competition. I have always been involved in some form of physical activity, beginning with team sports such as soccer and hockey when in school, moving onto swimming running and cycling as I got older, but in recent years I turned to adventure racing to get my thrills. Adventure races are multisport events and can include all sorts of challenges, such as abseiling, navigation, swimming, shooting, archery and puzzle-solving usually along with cycling, running and kayaking. The events I have participated in have taken many different formats, competing both as an individual and as part of a team. I have completed races from four hours in length through to a grueling 36 hours and even won a few prizes along the way. What I love most about adventure racing is the sense of achievement gained from competing. It can last for days after the event is over, especially after one of the more technical, longer races. For me, adventure racing was a chance to be a kid again and tap into that sense of adventure. There was also something nice and back-to-basics about it. It's hard to beat getting lost in the mountains at night and having to rely on your own resources and those of your team to get yourself out of sticky situations. It challenges the body and mind in ways that our sedentary lifestyles rarely allow nowadays. There is a serious lack of female competitors in the scene which is a shame as many of the women really shine in the longer endurance events where speed is less important. To compete successfully in adventure races requires a fairly solid fitness base and the training program needs to contain many elements that have to be worked on simultaneously, so it can be quite time consuming.

In August 2011, I was coming to the end of an epic adventure racing season. It had been my best yet – I had completed in over 10 races, with a number of podium finishes in both the team and individual events. I really felt like I was getting somewhere and was improving. People would soon be obliged to take me seriously as an athlete, something I had always wanted. Any sport would do! I seemed to be more of a jack of all trades, which was probably suited to adventure racing. When it came to different sports I was naturally good at getting the hang of things quickly but rarely excelled in anything I had tried. I had rarely won anything before plying my trade in multisport events. The previous year I hadn't even figured in the results and was just trying to survive. However, as I had built on my fitness base over the preceding winter, this year had seen significant improvements. I also tackled the infamous "Beast of Ballyhoura" adventure race for the first time in 2011. "The Beast," as it's fondly known by those who have competed in it, is a non-stop 36-hour adventure race which involves navigating hundreds of kilometers through day and night in a wild, mountainous area of Ireland spanning three counties known as the Ballyhoura region. The race covers many different disciplines and battling the "sleep monsters" is a big challenge. The sleep deprivation is particularly acute during The Beast as the race starts at the crack of dawn on a Saturday morning, with most competitors lucky to grab one or two hours sleep prior to the 3 a.m. bus journey to the start at 5 a.m. in a mystery location. The race is considered to be too short to stop for any meaningful sleep by the hardcore competitors who go straight through the night. Lightweight teams like ours might take a five minute nap up against a wall or on a wet patch of grass when the fatigue becomes unbearable and falling asleep on the bike becomes a very real danger. In 2011 we finished this race in the middle of the pack, which I considered a big achievement for me and my team. There is a huge buzz that comes from surviving and completing a course like that and I was as high as a kite for a week after it.

However, there was more going on than adventure racing in the summer of 2011. With much trepidation on my part, my husband and adventure racing teammate, Cormac, and I were trying for a baby. It wasn't that my biological clock was ticking particularly loudly but I felt I couldn't put it off any longer. I wasn't getting any younger and neither was he, claiming he didn't want to be too old to be able to enjoy the experience of raising a son or daughter. I knew a lot of people in their late thirties who had been having problems even conceiving, and frankly, was starting to worry myself that I might have problems as we had been trying for a couple of months and nothing seemed to be happening. "If you stopped all that running around and gave yourself half a chance you might have more success", my mother helpfully volunteered when I talked to her about it. This was not appealing to me at all. Racing was such a buzz and a passion of mine, even defining who I was to an extent, I panicked at the idea I might have to give it all up to even get pregnant! Not to mention the elephant in the room – what the hell was I going to do when I did get pregnant? How could I stop?

I didn't know anything about exercise and pregnancy at this point, but by and enlarge what I did know wasn't good. Comments by friends and material I had read rang through my head. "You'd better give up running just in case," one friend, and passionate hill runner, was told by her GP. "Easy swimming is fine" another suggested to me when I voiced my concerns or "Go for brisk walks every day instead". "What?" This was not what I wanted to hear! Brisk walking was not going to produce the levels of endorphins I was clearly addicted to. This kind of advice was all well and good for someone without my love for physical activity, but I wondered what all the elite athletes at the other end of the scale do? I was sure the likes of Paula Radcliffe and Sonia O'Sullivan didn't stop training during their pregnancies. Surely they didn't just swap running 100 miles a week for easy walks and gentle swimming. I thought I had heard somewhere that Paula in fact had run a marathon when seven months pregnant in an amazing time and trained right through her pregnancies, and I knew Sonia had won bronze in the world cross country championships three months after giving birth! I wondered how these women knew what to do. I decided that elite athletes were probably privy to specialist coaches who knew how hard one could train during pregnancy and just after birth.

There was another thing that was worrying me. I knew of numerous friends and family members that had abandoned life as they knew it when their first baby had come along. I'm talking about girls who were both recreational and committed athletes, their training falling by the wayside when baby arrived. When I questioned them as to why they weren't participating in sport any more as they had done pre baby I was told "your priorities totally change" and "I just simply didn't have the time". Not good. A good friend was giving me a lift one day and we were discussing the baby issue. He had two himself, one two-year-old and one six months old. During the course of the conversation I told him I thought I wanted to have baby. He sighed and informed me in a resigned tone, "Look, kids are great, don't get me wrong. But you know all that running around and racing you and Cormac always do? Well you can say goodbye to that for starters. You won't be doing any of that anymore. I can't even get out of the house for an hour to go for a jog". I was pretty gutted to hear this. I wanted to tell him it was his own fault for not prioritising his fitness or interest in sport, but how could I? Maybe he was right! What the hell did I know? I silently vowed to prove him wrong. I think that while listening to all these people what terrified me the most was that an all-encompassing feeling would suddenly come over me and I wouldn't actually *want* to partake in physical activity as I had done. Being a pretty competitive person I was worried I would lose the edge, or worse, the desire to compete anymore. Aside from this massive mental shift I was also worried about not having the time to do the training to compete. I was really worried that I wouldn't be able to do anything when I had to mind a small baby. I talked to Cormac about my concerns for both of us and we decided that we wouldn't allow it to happen to us. But really neither of us had a clue as to whether it would or not. I think this was my biggest fear about getting pregnant. Sport defined so much about my life and who I was. I really was scared that when I became pregnant and baby came along that that would be the end of it all.

To alleviate my worrying about this, I decided to take a proactive approach and investigate what information was available about women and exercise during pregnancy. I'd have to get through that phase first in relatively good physical condition and then I could worry about finding the time to exercise with the baby afterwards. I made a decision to keep doing as much exercise as possible through my pregnancy – should it ever happen. I reckoned I'd need that to keep me sane for starters. I also wanted to be informed about what was safe to do as I knew the minute I got pregnant my mother and God knew who else would be on my back telling me I should take it really easy or give it all up. My first port of call was of course Google and an Internet search to see what information I could find. Word combinations such as "athlete" and "pregnancy" and "exercise" yielded results with wildly different advice. Everyone who wrote anything seemed to have an opinion and I could not believe how polarised some of these views were. There seemed to be precious little in the way of good advice for recreational athletes like me that wasn't extremely conservative. When I tried to Google "*elite* athlete" and "pregnancy" or "exercise" I found even less.

The great mystery. I knew the information must be out there and competitive athletic women must be following some sort of training programs when pregnant, but any concrete reference to what they were doing remained elusive. During one of my searches I did find one PowerPoint presentation with some interesting advice. It described a study on elite pregnant athletes exercising up to five hours a day with no detrimental effects. Frustratingly, however, there were no references to back this up. Just some words on a PowerPoint slide. I also tried to find the author of the presentation to no avail. It seemed to be a dark art this exercise-during-pregnancy lark. But at least I knew there were women out there doing a significant amount of exercising when pregnant.

At this point I put the brakes on the Google searching and decided to try a different tack. There was just too much unreliable information on the Internet. I wanted to be more selective. As a scientist, and also a veterinarian, I decided the best approach would be to conduct my own scientific literature review to look for information in good robust peer-reviewed articles from a range of physiology and medical journals. The results produced less conflicting views on exercise during pregnancy, but by and large the suggestions were still quite conservative. The American College of Obstetricians and Gynecologists (ACOG) were widely quoted in the papers I came across. ACOG recommend that pregnant women who are free of any complications follow the "American College of Sports Medicine-Centers for Disease Control and Prevention" general guidelines for physical activity. They recommend women engage in 30 minutes or more of moderate physical activity per day on most days of the week at all stages of pregnancy. This was something concrete and, although conservative in the amount of exercise, at least they specified *moderate* which meant that the exercise should be "somewhat hard and relatively taxing".

Overall, I was astonished to find there has actually been so little in the way of research and the effects of exercise on pregnant women and their unborn babies over the last 20 or 30 years. I came across one recently written article that flagged this. The author suggested that it was because such research is highly contentious and even deemed unethical in some cases. Any research on pregnant women which forced them to exercise might put them or their babies at risk. A big might with no solid grounds I had discovered, but, as I quickly learned, the precautionary principle is applied across the board when it comes to pregnancy. Any woman who has ever undergone a pregnancy will know this to be true, not just when it comes to exercise, everything from supplements to medicines to foods and drink, anything that has not been conclusively proven to be totally harmless – well you better not.

Research to investigate the effects of high intensity exercise on the fetus appeared to be particularly fraught with ethical complications. The number of studies investigating it could nearly be counted on one hand, while the number of participants in each study on two! It is worth mentioning that none of these studies reported any ill effects on either mother or fetus and there was no evidence to indicate that exercise at higher intensities produces any harmful effects at all. I was particularly interested in this fact. One of the most common pieces of advice I encountered was that you should back substantially on the intensity of any exercise you are doing when pregnant. This is interesting considering there is absolutely nothing to support this in the literature.

I was beginning to understand why the approach taken when advising women about exercise levels and pregnancy was so conservative. It was clear that even though all the indicators pointed towards the benefits of exercise, no one wanted to be sued so backed off when providing advice. The literature review also gave me a clue as to why there was a vast amount of conflicting theories. As always, in the absence of good research, old wives tales prevail. As I trawled through the papers I eventually managed to tease out a few pertinent facts that would later give me some guidelines for my training. I found some good papers that basically stuck to the facts about what had and what had not been proven, as opposed to speculating about the dangers. One name kept cropping up during my review, that of an American medical doctor named James Clapp III. He has been involved in a lot of the medical research on exercise during pregnancy. Right from his earliest papers, he seemed to take an open-minded approach and clearly supported women in their quest to maintain a substantial exercise regime during pregnancy. Much of the work he has done was published during the 1990s and uncovers some very interesting and often surprising facts on the effects of exercising during different stages of pregnancy. Having a scientific background I'm very much concerned with the burden of proof so was happy to discover that a huge amount of the conservative advice that was in the general public domain was actually based on the precautionary principle and precious little on fact. I might not have had much to go on after this brief review but at least I had failed to unearth a single piece of robust literature to tell me to stop or reduce the levels of exercise I was currently participating in should I fall pregnant.

It was around the time I was competing in The Beast that I discovered track cycling existed in Ireland. I had wanted to try it since watching the Beijing Olympics in 2008, particularly on an indoor wooden banked velodrome. What a buzz it must be to feel the centrifugal forces as one powered around the steepest part of the banking in the middle of a race. I found it amazing that all these British athletes had suddenly come out of the woodwork and were winning medals on the track left right and centre. I was particularly fascinated when I heard about Rebecca Romero. Previously having competed as an Olympic rower, this amazing athlete had hardly sat on a bike before converting to the track four years previously and was now winning Olympic medals in her new discipline. I was blown away by this as I had assumed that track cycling was something you had to have been practicing since childhood to perform at this level. "Not at all", my kiwi brother-in-law, Alistair, informed me when Cormac and I were on a trip to New Zealand in January 2011, "Do you want to give it a go?" I could hardly believe my luck at this unforeseen opportunity. We had, in a rare moment of sanity, decided to escape the Irish winter and were on a two month trip to visit all our relatives in the southern hemisphere. We had stopped off in Invercargill, an agricultural market town at the bottom of the South Island of New Zealand, a place most backpackers go out of their way to avoid when on an NZ odyssey. "You have what here?", I asked in disbelief the day I arrived, "a proper 250m indoor velodrome?" This was pretty unbelievable – after all the town and greater surrounds had a population of a mere 50,000, and from what I could see most of these were sheep or deer farmers. There wasn't even a velodrome in the capital Auckland, for God's sake! "Yea, a bunch of local cycling enthusiasts got a campaign together and the Invercargill Licensing Trust (ILT) supplied the 8 million dollars required to build it", Alistair informed me. It turned out all the profits from alcohol and establishments that sell it in Invercargill go back into the community via the ILT and are used to fund sport, education and recreation in the area. I thought this was a brilliant idea, turning those profits into something really positive for the community.

The next day we were scheduled to go and try the track. Alistair had booked us a private session. Before the session, he and his father Doug brought us on a tour of the hallway, where there hung a series of pictures of the velodrome at different stages of construction. Then it was down to business. We walked under the building and up a long curved ramp wheeling the fixed-wheel track bikes with us and emerged into what was the heart of the velodrome. Glossy, smooth, pale wooden walls that were alarmingly sheer in places surrounded us. It was so beautiful it took my breath away. I was transfixed by this fantastic perfect feat of construction. Simultaneously terrified and excited to get going, I did a couple of very shaky laps on the flat to start off with Alistair cycling beside me encouraging me to relax while I tried to get used to the sensation of riding a track bike. Track bikes are very simple machines in essence. They have a fixed wheel, which means you cannot stop pedaling or freewheel, and no brakes or gears. "Whatever you do, don't try to stop pedaling," Alistair instructed me, "or the saddle will whack you on the ass and you'll go over the handlebars!" Sound advice and a rock many a rookie rider has perished on. Once I was moving comfortably on the flat and had demonstrated an ability to stop, Alistair shouted at me "OK Sue, whenever you feel ready ride around on the blue!" The blue or "cote d'azure" as it's commonly known is a powder blue strip about 30 inches wide at a slightly more forgiving angle to the wooden walls – 30 degrees at its worst, compared to the terrifying 45 degrees where the wooden banking is at its steepest. Afraid to think about it, I immediately picked up the pace and managed to ride a few laps on the blue strip without falling off. "Right", Alistair lectured, "now try to relax a bit and whenever you feel ready move up onto the boards and ride around on the black". The "black" is a line that goes around the bottom of the track about one foot above the blue. I move onto the wooden part of the track and pick up the pace again much to Alistair's amusement – "Settle down Sue! You only need to be moving at 25kph to stay up on the boards!" "As if!" I think to myself riding as fast as I can, not believing him. Besides, I had absolutely no idea what 25kph felt like on a bike!

Things were under control for a lap or two and I was starting to think that perhaps this wasn't as hard as it looked. However, as always, pride comes before a fall and I made the fatal mistake of looking down instead of straight ahead, freaked out and next thing I knew the bike and I were crashing onto the ground at one of the corners after sliding down the banking. It was a slow enough fall but I managed to take a layer of skin off my elbow and discovered later I had also created an impressive bruise on my behind. I had a quick snivel and felt sorry for myself, pride more than anything momentarily wounded, along with the handlebars of the bike which were slightly bent on impact. Alistair's dad Doug reassured me and readjusted the bars and encouraged me to get back up on the bike as soon as I felt able. As I shakily pushed myself off the railings, Alistair rode around in front of me. "Stay on my wheel Sue no matter what, I promise I'll make sure you're going fast enough not to fall off, and for God's sake look ahead! Not down like last time!" Within 10 minutes, my fall forgotten, I was elated, flying around on the red (the sprinters line about two feet above the black) and loving the sensation. After about 15 minutes of non-stop pedaling I came down for a breather, completely on a high. Once I recovered, Alistair suggested I try a few laps at the top of the track now that I was riding with more confidence. With trepidation I worked my way up with each successive lap and eventually managed to ride within a foot of the railing at the top. For some reason, much to Alistair's amusement, I felt like I had to be moving even faster than before to stay up, even though he assured me the same speed is required no matter your position on the banking. I wasn't taking any chances. After four or five laps at this frantic pace I was totally exhausted but so proud of myself. The whole time I was up near the top I was terrified to look down to see how high up I was and maintained a rigid stare straight ahead. We finished the session with a short race which he let me win and I was delighted with myself, but also strangely deflated now that the experience was over. That's the end of that I realised – my track cycling career was going to be short lived.

Back in Ireland during the summer I recounted my experience in NZ wistfully to a friend of mine who is a passionate cyclist. "Sure we have a track in Dublin", she informed me, "It's on Sundrive road near the canal! Did you not know? It's not the best now mind you, an outdoor tarmac one and is a bit the worse for wear but it's a cycling track and the principles are the same". I couldn't believe it! I Goggled it immediately and discovered we did indeed have a track and what's more it had recently undergone a facelift – a bit of resurfacing, a new clubhouse and a club called Sundrive Track Team based there with a small but active cohort of people managing it. There were regular structured training sessions scheduled that riders could participate in after they participated in an "accreditation" – this was an instruction session lasting approximately two hours to ensure you were able to ride safely on the track. I also noticed there were details on the website of a women's training day organised for the following weekend, to try and encourage more females to participate in track racing. I could hardly believe my luck. The training day would involve a chance to try some of the different events that make up an Olympic Omnium – the 500m Time Trial, the Individual Pursuit, the Scratch and the Elimination Race. I had seen some of these events at a track carnival in Invercargill so had some idea what was involved although I couldn't say I understood many of the rules. The only prerequisite was that a track accreditation session had to be completed before coming to the training day. This normally took place once a month at Sundrive, and unfortunately I had missed the July window. I was desperate to get to the training day so taking a chance I wrote an email begging the guy in charge to somehow sort me out. With a bit of persistence and when he could see I was serious, he grudgingly agreed to allow me to gatecrash a special junior accreditation session which was running the morning of the training day, that very Saturday.

I was both nervous and excited when Saturday came around. It happened to be an absolutely beautiful day and I headed off early to make sure I had plenty of time. I could hardly believe my eyes when I saw the track – it was quite lovely, in a different way to the indoor velodrome. It was much longer (468m in total) as most outdoor tracks are and the tarmac banking with all its colored lines sloped gently up at the corners. Nowhere near as dramatic as the steep wooden walls in Invercargill but fantastic all the same. I could hardly believe that this had been in Dublin and I hadn't heard about it. The rest of the accreditation group consisted nearly entirely of pre-teen boys aged 10-12. I introduced myself to Hugh, the coach running the session as his "oversize" student, he was the person I had cajoled by email into letting me join in this session. I was feeling a bit conspicuous, sticking out like a sore thumb basically being about twice the size of most of the young lads but once we got moving and learning about track awareness, moving up the banking, overtaking safely and all the other skills involved I forgot about it. Track riding is quite technical to do safely and requires a different level of concentration to riding on the road. The outdoor track although a totally different experience to riding inside had a surprising number of similarities. I liked it! The women's training started up soon after the accreditation ended and we got to try our hand at all the different events that make up the Olympic Omnium.

First was the Scratch Race. The rules of this one were pretty straightforward. It involved a 10 km race and first over the line was the winner. Hugh, who was again coaching the session, told us that he didn't care what we did as long as we all tried something, anything at all, during the race, such as make an attack or chase someone down. I didn't really have a clue what he was talking about but decided to "attack". Unfortunately, being so green, I did this a bit too far out, attacking with 10 laps to go. I opened up a gap of about 100 m on the bunch and then after a minute or so started to notice how hard it was when you were riding without the shelter of the other riders. I stuck with the plan however and I pedaled on as hard as I could with gritted teeth. Needless to say I couldn't keep this up indefinitely and they caught me with two laps to go as I died. I did feel slightly ridiculous out there in front for all those laps. I consoled myself that I had tried something at least.

The Elimination Race was next. The last rider across the line at every lap is eliminated. I managed to hang in there until there were four laps to go, which at least wasn't too shameful. Next came an event I really wanted to try, the Individual Pursuit. This was the event in which I had watched Rebecca Romero ride to victory in, in the Beijing Olympics. There was something engaging about being pitted against another person in a frantic race to stay ahead of them, a true battle of mind body and determination. As I sat there clipped into my bike waiting to start I was an absolute bag of adrenalin – It was as though I were the one in the Olympics! I glanced over at my much younger, but more experienced opponent, with her pursuit bars and aero helmet and got another wave of the jitters. "Oh God, I'm going to vomit", I thought. Then we were off! I powered off as if my life depended on it. This meant a very fast first lap and at the one lap mark I was ahead of the other girl by about five meters. "The pressure is on me now", I thought, "I have to maintain my lead". I was starting to tire already having bolted too fast at the start. Prior to this, I had no idea the Pursuit is about a measured steady effort and the best riders often get slightly faster and stronger as the laps go on. I was entirely focused on the line I was riding round the track, watching the meter etchings ticking by - 100, 200, 300 meters. All I could hear was the wind and the sound of my own ragged breathing. Before I knew it, it was over – yet simultaneously it felt like the longest three minutes of exercise I ever did. I was weak afterwards and as I wobbled over to the fence I struggled to unclip from my pedals. Clutching the railings, I asked for my time. "2. 56," Hugh said. "Is that good?" I asked realising I hadn't a clue. "That's very good for a first time, especially in this wind," he answered, and looking a bit surprised added a second later "In fact it's excellent". Although I had seriously suffered I was delighted with myself.

The Pursuit was the highlight of my day. One of the best female riders at the track went next and she rode eight seconds faster than me. I was delighted with this too as I didn't see it as too much of an improvement on what I did. "I could probably knock eight seconds off my time, "I thought to myself, "if I had a decent bike, a set of pursuit bars and one of those fancy helmets!" And a bit of specific training and practice of course might help too. I got the first inkling that day that maybe this was something I could be good at. I went home that evening with a very sore backside from the unforgiving saddles on the rental bikes and a new obsession – track cycling. From then on I started to attend all the training sessions. I was finding ways to leave work early to be back in time for Wednesday night racing. I ditched my adventure racing training as I became obsessed with the track – the season was so short and I had missed most of it. I even gave up running as Hugh convinced me it slowed leg speed – which apparently was one of the most important strings to your bow as a track cyclist. Less than a month later, I competed in the National Track Championships which was a baptism of fire. The standard of rider was also out of sight for me. Two weeks after the Nationals I competed in the regional championships where I fared a bit better and won a bronze medal in the 500 meter Time Trial. I look back at a picture someone took of me on the podium that day and I don't think I ever valued a medal as much. Despite my fascination with the Pursuit, I seemed to be showing more promise at the sprinting events. I was naturally fast at standing starts, which really helps in short events like the 500TT. "You start like a man," Terry one of the coaches informed me, "and that's the best compliment I can give you!" I was delighted with myself and every time I did a 500TT I managed to knock another few fractions of a second off. After my bronze medal in the regional championships, with a time of 42.5 seconds, Hugh informed me, "I think with the right training you'll be able to go below 40 next year, and we'll see what you're made of after that". I was excited to think I might have that potential. A 39 second TT would have been enough for a safe gold in the regional Championship and what's more a podium finish in the Nationals. The outdoor record for the 500TT in Ireland currently stands at 38.5 seconds. I started to fantasize that someday in the next few years maybe I could claim this record. I have always been a bit of a dreamer!

Starting a new sport is so full of promise and excitement which I love. You have no idea of your potential and to challenge this and push the boundaries is so much fun. It was in these early days at the track that Orla Hendron, one of the other more experienced female track riders, said to me, "You should do the World Masters in Manchester. It's a great way to get free indoor track time." Orla herself had actually won a world title at the Masters in the points race in 2010. The World Masters Track Cycling Championships is open to anyone over the age of 35. It is a world championships largely for amateur athletes and people compete against others in their age group. The seed was sown. I started to imagine being on the boards in Manchester. I had seen this velodrome on TV, as it had been used for many major competitions. "I shouldn't even be thinking about this," the sensible side of my brain reasoned, "I'll be killed!" But I knew I would find a way to go. I talked to enough people who encouraged me with stories of being as green as me themselves and competing in previous years – it didn't take much to convince me that I should chance it. I started to hatch a plan.

When I ran the idea by Hugh, he tried initially to put me off as he knew it would be hard for me to be competitive and probably dangerous with my complete lack of technical indoor riding skills. However, once he realised how determined I was to go he became my number one supporter. "OK, you can borrow my wheels for starters. And my tools and pump and anything else you need. You'll have to practice visualising what's involved in a Flying 200 since you won't get a chance to do one indoors before the day, and I'll talk you through some strategies for the sprinting. The bunch races are dangerous if you're not used to them but if you really want to do one for God's sake do the Scratch Race rather than the Points Race – you've less chance of being killed in that one. I'll email you warm up sessions to do before each event." And so it went on.

However, a curveball was in store. In the midst of all this day-dreaming and planning my future as a track cyclist in September 2011, I got pregnant. I realised that there was something funny going on with my body while I was away at an international conference in Croatia. I was presenting some research on a new bacterial disease in the gills of salmon. Being a veterinarian who works primarily with fish, this was one of my areas of expertise. At the conference dinner on the night I arrived, there were vast arrays of delicious salads to choose from. I fell upon a plate piled with roasted aubergines bathed in olive oil. "Mmm, my favorite," I thought, as I helped myself to a generous portion. I got back to the table and proceeded to tuck in. After two or three mouthfuls of aubergine a wave of nausea came over me and I found myself retching. "What the hell?" I thought, "there must be something wrong with these". All of a sudden it hit me, maybe it wasn't the aubergines. "What if I'm pregnant?," I thought to myself. As soon as I said it, I kind of knew I had to be as that reaction to aubergines was so completely out of character. I didn't want to think about or deal with it. I decided to go into denial. After all, my period wasn't that long overdue, maybe only by a day or two. Or was it? After a few months of trying and failing to get pregnant earlier that year I had realised my monthly cycles were actually a week longer than the standard 28 days and my periods were actually 35 days apart. I did a quick calculation and realised I was on day 36. A few days later and no sign of monthly cycles arriving, I knew it was highly likely I was pregnant. After two or three false alarms in the previous six months and about 30 euros spent on pregnancy tests, I decided, now that I was for the first time pretty sure of my status, I would take a new approach – denial. "I'll worry about it when I get home," I thought. I had rented a bike for the week in Croatia and was trying to get in about 2 hours training on it every morning before the conference kicked off. I continued with this plan, trusting that I wasn't going to do the baby any harm at this stage, sure it was only a few cells. I wasn't even sure I was happy about being pregnant. How was this going to affect my plans for the World Masters? I did another quick calculation and realised I would be about seven weeks pregnant while competing. I really had my heart set on it and didn't want to give up the dream. I decided that denial was, indeed, probably the best and most productive approach to take for the moment. Once I got home I took up my pregnancy and exercise literature review again in earnest.

SUSIE MITCHELL

THE QUEST FOR KNOWLEDGE

On my return home I immediately renewed my scientific literature review of exercise during pregnancy. My first discovery was that research investigating the safety of exercise during pregnancy was pretty thin on the ground up until the 1980s. Only anecdotal reports of the occasional elite athlete who continued exercising throughout her pregnancy without incident were available. Then in 1985, due to rising pressure from both doctors and exercising mothers, the American College of Obstetricians and Gynecologists (ACOG) published a set of guidelines and contraindications to exercise during pregnancy. This was the first published text dealing with the issue. Unfortunately for me, even though they were advocating exercise during pregnancy, I felt it was a highly conservative set of guidelines, and these guidelines seemed to be formulated based largely on the theoretical risks to the mother and fetus as opposed to actual risks. The "just in case" approach. Doctors around the world breathed a collective sigh of relief. Or at least, those who has been troubled by the fact that they didn't really have any advice on exercise guidelines for pregnant women did. Having said that, many still continued in the same vein, advising the mother take it easy and do little or nothing. The principles that the ACOG guidelines were based on may have been very conservative but doctors didn't care! At last they had a get out clause and couldn't be liable should anything happen to the women they were advising about exercise during pregnancy. So, sadly, instead of providing advice based on their own experience, knowledge of human physiology and instinct many resorted to referring to the ACOG guidelines. This is understandable. Unfortunately, not just doctors but other healthcare providers are in constant fear of being held responsible or liable should something go wrong, especially during a pregnancy, so it's clear as to why these conservative guidelines were embraced. The ACOG guidelines were revised and updated to some degree in the 1990s taking much of the research that had subsequently occurred into pregnancy and exercise into account, but still remained largely conservative, basically advising women to dramatically reduce the intensity and duration of their exercise, as well as suggesting only certain types of exercise might be suitable during pregnancy, such as stationary cycling, swimming or walking.

This was all very depressing for me, but at least I was getting to the root of why this conservative advice was there and was beginning to understand the lack of support for people who wanted to continue with their normal exercise regime. Thankfully, over the course of my research, I was heartened to discover I was not alone in my desire to continue with my normal training. I came across some physically active women who maintained vigorous exercise regimes right through pregnancy. I met some of these women, got in touch with others via email and heard about what others did through word of mouth. While it wasn't easy to access the information, there was a network out there. Many of these women were fortunate enough to have been supported by more open-minded healthcare providers or coaches, but some did it alone in the face of advice to the contrary. They seemed to be largely making it up as they went along, based on common sense and how they felt at the time.

Interested in establishing what the general opinion on the matter was, I quizzed everyone I met informally on their general thinking on exercise and pregnancy. I discovered people's opinions were generally strong and extremely polarized. By and large Irish people seemed to have pretty conservative views on exercise during pregnancy. There was definitely a notion that it's good to do some exercise during pregnancy but most people thought the quantity of and intensity should be dramatically reduced, while some activities should be avoided altogether, such as running and cycling. "There has to be a different slant on this", I said to Cormac after one long afternoon listening to my in-laws opinions. "Because if there isn't I quite possibly will go mad over the next few months!"

It was with much trepidation and this in mind that I went to visit my consultant obstetrician for the first time at 18 weeks pregnant, wondering what his views would be. I was quietly optimistic. I had heard on the grapevine that he was the best in the business, but pretty tough and had a no nonsense approach. Apparently, when someone had complained about their morning sickness to him he said, without too much empathy, "What do you expect? You're pregnant..!" He definitely wasn't a hand-holder. So in I went in to the clinic and when my scan and blood pressure measurement were out of the way, I took a deep breath before making my case for exercise. "I do a lot of exercise, particularly cycling and some running, go to the gym and so on and was wondering if..." At this point he interrupted me without blinking and said "Keep doing whatever you're doing until you can do it no longer." It was like music to my ears! He didn't seem too concerned about specifics and I didn't ask anymore as I practically danced out the door delighted. The following weekend I was out for a long Sunday spin with my club. I was telling Pat, one of the ladies in the group, about my experience with my obstetrician. She asked me his name and we discovered he had delivered her two babies about 20 years previously. "At the time I was playing a lot of tennis", she told me, "and he told me the same thing. He's great. I played and competed until I was about 6 months pregnant." I asked if she felt she wasn't up to playing any longer after that. "You must be joking!" she said, "I only stopped because no one would play against me once my bump started showing. I love playing at the net you see, and my opponents were all afraid they would hit me with a tennis ball and do some damage!" We laughed at that. It was great to hear that my obstetrician has been advising women to keep up their exercise regime for decades. He had obviously realised through years of experience that his mums-to-be who exercised at a significant level did much better during pregnancy and birth, and that it certainly didn't do them any harm.

As I continued my literature search to investigate what I could and couldn't do during pregnancy, I found James Clapp's name kept popping up over and over. An American medical doctor, he appeared to have been involved in most of the research that interested me. I was lucky enough at that point to stumble across the fact that he had actually written a book about pregnancy and exercise, which summarized all the important findings from his research over the years. I ordered a copy from the United States immediately. I couldn't believe it but it wasn't on sale in Ireland or the UK – thank God for Amazon. Once I got my hands on the book, I devoured it. It turned out he was the first person to carry out any significant research into the effects of exercising through pregnancy. He had started his investigations in the late 70s and subsequently went on to do much of the interesting and relevant research into the effect of exercise during pregnancy on both the mother and the baby in the following years, and continues to be involved in such research to this day. His first step in the early years was to study the effects of exercise on pregnancy in sheep rather than using human subjects. Using pregnant ewes he put them through their paces on a specially designed sheep treadmill and investigated the effects of strenuous exercise on both maternal body temperature and blood flow to the placenta. These were the two factors people were most concerned about with exercise during pregnancy. Maybe it's because of my veterinary background and that I used to work with sheep, but I found his descriptions of his first experiments hilarious. To get the sheep to stay on the treadmill with all the measuring equipment attached to her, they had to surround the moving belt with a plywood pen. As Dr Clapp ramped up the speed of the treadmill, he found that absolutely nothing happened to the sheep's heart rate, her blood pressure, respiration or the rate of blood flow to the placenta. She simply looked calmly at the doctor over the top of the pen, chewing the cud. He doubled the speed and could hear the treadmill running but there was still no effect on her physiological parameters. When he finally stood up and looked over the edge down into the pen he discovered the ewe was straddling the belt, balanced precariously on one toe from each foot on the quarter inch rail at each side of the moving belt as it flew past under her. Outwitted by a sheep! After that, he modified the treadmill so the ewe couldn't cheat.

Once he managed to get the sheep engaged in strenuous exercise Dr Clapp found maternal body temperature rose significantly as expected and blood flow to the placenta was reduced to 50% of normal. Even though both the responses were dramatic and, in theory, potentially harmful, the unborn lambs handled the stress very well even after an hour of strenuous exercise. The outcome of the study showed the fetus effectively tolerated these stresses very well and did so well into late pregnancy. This early experiment really was the first evidence of the body's ability to adapt to exercise during pregnancy. Other investigators repeated these types of experiments and measured more detailed parameters. They exercised sheep at high intensity near their maximal capacities for protracted periods. Even though, again, there was a decrease in blood flow to the fetus and placenta in the sheep they studied, there were no ill effects whatsoever to the fetal lambs. I was really pleased to see the results of this research. I knew sheep weren't humans but I felt the physiology would definitely be somewhat comparable to our own. It certainly made sense to me that we and other animals would have coping mechanisms in place to deal with strenuous activity during pregnancy – no species would be able to survive without it in the natural world. Tigers don't give their prey a special dispensation because they're pregnant. Prey animals such as gazelles and wildebeest still have to be able to take flight to ensure the survival of their young when pregnant themselves. We might not have the need to engage in strenuous activity to survive in modern day life but our predecessors in the evolution of the species (*Homo erectus*) did. They were always on the move, reputedly running up to thirty miles a day while hunting wild animals. I reasoned that our species wouldn't be here today if pregnant *Home erectus* females couldn't hack it. The evidence was slowly mounting for me that it was safe to push the body while pregnant.

While the results of the sheep studies suggest that exercise even at high intensities is acceptable, some differences in species were likely to apply, so Dr Clapp moved on to investigate similar parameters in human subjects willing and open-minded enough to participate in his studies. Principally, he studied runners and aerobics instructors, due to the relatively intense nature of their workouts and the fact that they would frequently exercise for long periods. During these studies he also selected a control group of healthy, but non-exercising, women. He not only followed these two cohorts of women while pregnant but also followed their babies post-partum, and continues to do so to this day to monitor the long-term effects on children born to exercising moms. He reported his findings from all of his experiments to date in detail in his book and I relished every page.

Because of my background in veterinary medicine, I had some knowledge of the general physiological changes that occur in the body during pregnancy. What I found particularly interesting about Dr Clapp's book, however, were the details of how the body uses these normal physiological adaptations to allow us to engage in strenuous exercise. For example, when pregnant, you sweat at a lower temperature. Body temperature rises with strenuous exercise so this early sweating mechanism can help counteract this. He also went on to describe how many of the training effects that occur in the body in response to regular physical exercise actually mirror what happens with pregnancy, and therefore the two could complement each other. I knew this to be true as I had personally observed that as I became fitter over the previous few years I found I sweated a lot earlier and more during training sessions.

Another interesting detail he described was the phenomenon whereby exercising at different stages of your pregnancy can stimulate specific extra changes and adaptations which allow you to exercise more efficiently when in the pregnant state. It seemed to me that the body is a very clever machine indeed, and these adaptations to allow us to exercise efficiently when pregnant are hardly there by accident. We evolved that way for a reason. Finally, by describing the physiological changes associated with each trimester the book provided a great insight into explaining the side effects we feel as pregnancy progresses and to know what is normal and what to expect your body to feel like when exercising during these different stages. I will talk more about these adaptations in the next chapter.

Aside from Dr Clapp, who quickly became my main guide on exercise and pregnancy, I also came across a researcher in Holland who had written a few very positive papers in recent years about the benefits of exercise during pregnancy. I decided to email him and ask his advice and for a copy of one or two of his papers. He was actually the first person I told I was pregnant and knew even before Cormac! I figured he wouldn't tell anyone I knew as he was safely tucked away in Amsterdam. My letter to him was as follows:

Dear Professor,
I am emailing you as I would really like a copy of your article entitled "Physical Activity and Pregnancy: Cardiovascular Adaptations, Recommendations and Pregnancy Outcomes", published in 2010 in Sports Medicine.

I am a pretty competitive amateur athlete (mostly cycling - track, cycloX) and plan to train throughout my pregnancy - I have been doing so far and all is going well. In fact am performing very well in the last few weeks and feel great for it, and the baby appears healthy also. The problem I am encountering is that is its very hard to get good unbiased scientific data on what you can and can't do when pregnant, and people who give advice tend to do so using the precautionary principle, the "just in case" approach - for instance the recommendation to exercise only at sub maximal intensity below 70% max HR - this doesn't come from any scientific studies or data that I can see, yet it is quoted everywhere!

It is frustrating as, being a scientist myself, I want to know the facts, what has been studied, what has been shown to cause damage to the fetus etc. I have decided to do my own literature review on the available information as a result. I just found your article on-line and thought it would be a good place to start. I hope you can send me a copy. Also, any other papers you have published on pregnancy and exercise would be greatly appreciated. The way the attitudes to pregnancy and exercise have shifted over the last number of years, I wouldn't be surprised if the advice is to run several marathons while pregnant at some stage in the future! I would love to volunteer for a study to try and further the knowledge in this area, and I'm sure there are many others out there like me. Only problem is trying to find researchers willing to take the chance that they might end up with a bad result if pushing pregnant athletes too hard - and that's understandable too! It's a bit of a catch 22.

His reply came a day later, as follows:

"Dear Susie,
Here is the article. I attach a few others, arguing in favour of physical activity during pregnancy. If you are young, healthy, and athletic, just continue what you have been doing all along.

Just two advices:
Listen up to your body. You will feel it signalling eventually when running is perhaps not best way to work out anymore in the last trimester. But then change activity. My wife was doing cross country skiing (skating) a few weeks before giving birth, but wouldn't run anymore since it felt unpleasant. She would bring our first one in a bike trailer to the day-care. My mother cycled to day care with one kid in front, one on the back, one in her tummy, but that was in the Netherlands, a very bike-friendly environment.

Choose activities where (accidental) impact is rare. I would advise against kick-boxing, down-hill skiing. I would be choosy with regard to the type of biking. Sounds obvious perhaps, but you would be amazed ...

Wish you all the best; isn't it wonderful, giving life, the very meaning of life!"

Once I read his mail I felt that this was probably the best two pieces of sensible advice I was going to get off anyone: Listen to your body and avoid sports with a risk of blunt abdominal trauma. Looking back they were probably the two most important pieces of advice I received during my entire pregnancy and post-partum, and I have re-iterated it to anyone who asks me about exercise and pregnancy. I also reluctantly realised that his advice on biking made sense and I would probably have to shelve the mountain bike for a few months – given the amount of accidents I had had on it.

I really liked his email. There was nothing reflecting the 'just in case' approach, just common sense and encouragement. With an active wife and mother, he clearly had a good understanding of a woman who needs exercise as part of her daily routine. The last line of his mail also struck a chord: "Wish you all the best; isn't it wonderful, giving life, the very meaning of life!" I was still somewhat in denial mode I wasn't really thinking like this about pregnancy. It did give me an inkling that something big was happening, but it was going to take me a while to get my head around the life changing experience element. Of course, at that stage I really had no idea what was in store.

Armed with the Professor's advice and Dr Clapp's research, I decided to forge ahead and trust my body. Being used to all sorts of training I knew how it felt to exercise comfortably in my aerobic zone, knew what intense exertion felt like, and knew how nearly vomiting after a session when pushing my limits felt. So I knew what felt normal for exercise and trusted my body would let me know if I was doing anything that was not good for the baby. I continued my training programme for the Masters unfettered, which at this stage mostly involved short speed drills, improving my leg speed and perfecting my standing starts. I was also doing some intense sessions behind the derny (a motorbike used for pacing during track cycling to optimize power output at high speeds). All this felt OK and although I was a bit nervous, on the Professor's advice, I trusted my body.

October 2011 rolled around pretty quickly and it was finally time to travel to the World Track Masters Championships in Manchester. To my surprise, with all the worry about whether I should even be going, I nearly missed the ferry by sleeping in the morning of departure. I fell out of the bed at 8.15am to make a 9am ferry with the port a 15 minute drive away. I was under pressure. It was a good thing that I had packed all the bags the night before. My husband helped fire all my gear, including two bikes, into my roomy estate car and I was on the road by 8.30am. I screeched up to departures and was the last car onto the boat, driving on as they were raising the ramp behind me! I had noticed that sleeping a lot more can be a side-effect of early pregnancy, so that had probably been responsible for the ill-timed sleep in.

Thanks to my recently purchased sat-nav, which had proved useless in Ireland but came into its own once I entered the UK, the rest of the journey was uneventful. After a few hours drive I arrived at the Manchester velodrome and entered the track center. The whole place was electric and alive, full of people and noise, and I immediately had some serious butterflies. Crews of people from all over the world were milling around, from women in their mid-30s to elderly men in their mid-70s. The Irish group had a small area cordoned off for warming up and storing gear and a few familiar faces were already there, which was reassuring. Competitions were in full swing by the time I arrived as I had elected to only do three events in the middle of the week – the Scratch Race, the Match Sprint and, what I felt would be the big one for me, the 500m TT. I had hoped that I would improve on my time of 42.5 seconds achieved on the outdoor track during the Regional Championships. Generally as a rule of thumb, due to reduced wind resistance and friction, people tend to ride faster indoors in this event.

The women's 35-39 year old 500m TT was going to be the morning after I arrived. I managed to squeeze in a practice session in the velodrome that evening so I had at least been able to remind myself what it felt like to ride indoors. However, the practice sessions were so busy there was no chance of getting in a proper 500m effort. Just staying upright and avoiding being taken out of it by some crazy European was an achievement in itself. Nevertheless, I was comfortable both on the bike and on the boards by the time the session ended.

The following morning I was scheduled as the first rider to go in the 500m TT. This honor was imposed on me as I had never posted a time indoors in any other competition. The slowest rider goes first. I felt sick with nerves. The air was stifling inside the velodrome and there were bright lights shining on me from every angle – or at least that's what it felt like. I clambered onto the bike after the official fixed it in the starting gate and the countdown from 50 seconds began. During practice sessions at Sundrive I had found that the best way to get out of the gate quickly was to use my ears instead of watching the countdown on the clock in front of me. I would listen to the beeps which occur simultaneously to the last 5 seconds on the countdown timer, then wait to hear the puff of air as the hydraulic arm from the gate released my bike, then go all out. It is best to be a little slow leaving the gate, as jumping the gun could be disastrous for your standing start. I was confident my little trick of listening for the hiss of air was foolproof as it had consistently worked for me in practice sessions at home. What I hadn't counted on was the extra noise in the velodrome and my state of hyper arousal as I sat out the countdown. Not to mention the fact that this gate was a bit different and actually made an additional noise a split second before the hydraulic arm released the bike. This was my downfall. With the (wrong) hiss, totally charged on adrenalin, I threw my entire body weight forward and stomped on the pedals expecting to explode out of the gate. For a horrible second though nothing happened. I was just stuck there, over the handlebars, legs straining against non-yielding pedals – it was like everything was happening in slow motion. "You've gone too early, got stuck in the gate!", I realised. in what could have only been a split-second. I felt defeated and disappointed before I even started. Then the gate released and I lurched forward in a pretty haphazard manner, my legs already burning from the wasted strain they had been put under. I quickly refocused and gave it everything I had but the fluidity I normally felt as I built up speed from the standing start wasn't there. I pushed as hard as I could right through to the end and looked up at the clock. My heart sank when I saw my time of 42.45 – hardly better than I had done on the outdoor track a few weeks previously. I was devastated. One chance is all you got at this level. As it turned out I placed eight out of eleven riders so it wasn't too bad considering, but I had hoped for so much more. I texted Hugh to tell him the bad news. Ever positive, he found the silver lining "Well you will never do that again" he texted back, "and next time it might really matter!" I grudgingly had to accept he was probably right, and it was a lesson well learned.

The Scratch Race was next and the race I was most nervous about – I had never ridden a bunch race on an indoor track. Nevertheless, I decided that I really wanted to do it and I wouldn't take any unnecessary risks so it would be alright – or so I reasoned. There were about twenty girls in the race as two age groups were combined to make the race more interesting. This made me a little more nervous than I had initially been but I decided to go ahead regardless. The race was a pretty short 5km so the pace was blistering right from the gun and my mouth was as dry as sandpaper with nerves (or maybe that was another side effect of early pregnancy!). I made the mistake of not getting into a great position at the start so was riding about two thirds of the way back in the bunch. I had a number of opportunities where the pace temporarily slowed and the group opened up a bit but I felt, given my state, it would have been downright reckless to go for the gaps that were created and I'd be pushing my luck – I had promised myself beforehand that all I wanted to do was survive the race and not get dropped. I was unfortunately boxed in so couldn't go over the top of the bunch either. In the end I crossed the line in around tenth position which was a pretty good result for a first timer erring on the side of caution due to an extra passenger. I was thrilled with myself and absolutely ecstatic after it. That day was also my birthday which made it all the more special. My present to myself, I thought.

 The final competition I entered was the Match Sprint. This was an event that required something more than fitness, strength and speed. Cunning, a certain attitude and experience play an equally important role in head-to-head sprinting. It's like a game of cat and mouse and all about getting the jump on your opponent. You have to have all kinds of skills to be a good sprinter. It helps, for instance, if you can stare intimidatingly at your opponent, ride looking over your shoulder, bluff and trick the other rider into jumping too early where you can take advantage of their mistakes. Every Match Sprint is different and unpredictable. I was a complete greenhorn and had none of these skills. Many of the other Irish riders were looking at me like I had two heads for even trying it. Something about it though lured me in. I had participated in this event in the Irish Track National's a few weeks previously, where I was made a show of by a more experienced rider. Instead of discouraging me, it left me hungry for more.

To be matched with an opponent for the sprinting every competitor has to do a Flying 200. This is a 200m time trial from a moving or flying start and was something I had never done on an indoor track. It is pretty technical and can be difficult to get right, as you have to accelerate at exactly the right time and hold your line on the track at full speed. Due to my lack of experience, I was forced to practice solely using visualisation. Hugh had emailed me a description of what I should be doing at every stage of each lap during the wind up and then during the actual 200m. I walked around the center of the velodrome muttering the instructions to myself, trying to see myself up there on the boards. Although I had been dubious, the visualization worked pretty well and I posted a time of 13.87 – a pretty good first ever attempt. This time matched me against an American girl who was a very experienced sprinter. As her Flying 200 had been nearly a second faster than mine I knew I had to try getting a good jump on her if I was to have any chance of beating her. As we circled the track I tried moving her around a bit, forcing her up on the banking then slowing down. Unfortunately, I had neither the technical skill nor the know how to do anything significant and when I tried to get the jump on her she was ready and came around me with 50m to go and comfortably beat me. All in all I really enjoyed it though and it gave me a taste for what I could potentially do with a bit of appropriate training and practice.

At the end of the few days I came away from Manchester with an overriding sense of satisfaction and silently thanked God and anyone else who was listening that I had gotten through it pregnant but unscathed. I was already thinking about next October. I knew the Masters were to be held again in Manchester and I was planning to return with the intention of seriously improving my performance and perhaps even winning a medal. I had done the math in my head. The baby was due on the 23rd of May which would give me about four to five months to recover and get back up to speed. I had no idea if this would be possible but I made a decision to give it my best shot. To do this, I knew it was even more important now that I continue to train during my pregnancy. There was no way starting from scratch next May or June would be sufficient to have me in shape to compete. When I came home I faced into the same uncertainly about what I could and couldn't do. Even though I was now more confident that the training I was doing was probably working, I still hadn't really worked any specifics out. As well as continuing to review scientific papers, I ordered a couple of general books on the internet to see what was out there besides Dr Clapp's scientific book. While there was an abundance of books on yoga and Pilates during pregnancy, there weren't actually many general books available on exercise and pregnancy. In the end I purchased five different books which turned out to be nearly identical to each other in content. Again, they echoed the conservative approach that had become the norm when providing guidelines for exercising pregnant women, and used the ACOG guidelines as their cornerstone piece of advice. At this point when I sat back to reflect on it all I really started to feel for all the other women out there like me, for whom sport and competition was a large part of their lives and helped define who they were. I came to the sad conclusion that all these books I had purchased, and many more like them, were all the same. They were supposed to be providing advice for pregnant women on appropriate exercise regimes but were too conservative and limited. I realised it was impossible they could be otherwise - they needed to avoid liability in the event that someone following their guidelines lost a baby, or something equally awful.

As I reflected on this I reached a decision. *I* would write a book! The book I had been looking for but couldn't find. The book I would have liked to read now, but didn't exist. I would include important facts on the physiology of pregnancy and exercise based on scientific research. And I would tell my story, describe my journey. Not tell women what they should or shouldn't do. But outline the facts and tell them what I did, how it felt and how it worked for me. I hoped my book would allow women take an alternative approach, and make up their own minds about what exercise they could do when pregnant and post-partum. I decided to include details of all the training I did right throughout my pregnancy, the racing I did during pregnancy and how I felt post-partum and my return to full fitness, as it happened. I also had another inkling of an idea. Pregnancy is an amazing life changing experience in itself, and I already believed you could probably use this unique physiological state to your advantage as an athlete. I imagined that training while pregnant would provide all sorts of benefits. As pregnancy places the body under physiological stress, it was like an opportunity to train at altitude. For instance, I knew from reading Dr Clapp's book that your hematocrit post-partum, once your blood volume returns to normal (usually after about four to six weeks), is increased by approximately 20%. Who needs EPO I thought. Those early weeks post-partum might not be a time when you will post new personal bests, but I reckoned with an aerobic boost like that it's an ideal time to regain any fitness lost during pregnancy. I believed deep down it might in fact be possible to alter your outcomes in fitness and competition post pregnancy if you optimized your training program while pregnant. In the next few chapters I am going to discuss the physical, mechanical, hormonal, circulatory and respiratory effects that happen at different stages and suggest how, with the addition of training, that can lead to a better, stronger and faster athlete post-partum.

Stories abound of women from all sporting disciplines who not only come back to full competitive fitness after pregnancy, but who come back stronger and post new personal records. The benefits seem to be not only physiological, but psychological. Having said this, at the same time I am aware that pregnancy is a different experience for every woman and can also be different too, depending on which child they are having – first second or sixth. What I did may not be suitable for everyone, but by writing my story I wanted to at least provide an alternative approach for those out there like me, who love exercise and competition and want to continue through pregnancy and beyond.

FIRST TRIMESTER – IN DENIAL

As I mentioned previously, I figured out I was pregnant when at a conference in Split, a city in Croatia. The conference was a gathering of people working in the area of fish diseases, and happens every two years, called the EAFP or "The European Association of Fish Pathologists". This is about as exciting as it sounds to anyone not interested in fish diseases. I was going to present some findings from my PhD which I had worked on part time and just completed, and had been looking forward to getting away for a week in the sun. I was also looking at the trip as an opportunity to do some "warm weather training" – it would make a nice change to ride a bike in the warm sunshine I thought. I had arranged a bike rental for the duration so I could continue to train for the Masters in Manchester in October. The weather was stunning there and it grew quite hot during the day, so I was up and out on my bike for an hour or two at 6.30am every morning. Little did I know on those first few mornings that my training was to be disrupted. When I gobbled down those few mouthfuls of chargrilled aubergines at the conference dinner and a wave of nausea engulfed me, I just knew. I felt, had I been a cartoon character, a light bulb would have flashed on over my head saying "Pregnant!" When I think back on it now, I had been feeling a little odd for the previous few days. On the bike I seemed to be getting out of breath a little sooner than expected and my heart rate was erratic. I had also felt a little dizzy when I got up in the morning. Yes, suddenly it all made sense.

I was surprised at how tired I felt during the first trimester of my pregnancy. I am normally so full of energy and usually active non-stop, requiring at most seven hours sleep a night. I had always been a night owl too, usually only turning in around midnight. Frankly, I had assumed a lot of people who had complained of being tired when pregnant were exaggerating and it wouldn't happen to me due to my naturally high energy levels. Well I was seriously wrong. I seemed to be alright during the daytime but once the clock struck 10pm, if I wasn't already horizontal in bed I had to crawl into the bedroom on hands and knees and slump under the covers. I found I needed about an extra hour or two sleep at least per night. The whole situation was probably not helped by having to wake up at least twice during the night to take a trip to the bathroom, no matter when I had peed last, or how little I had drunk prior to going to bed. My husband was wondering what was wrong with me. He had always been tucked up in bed before me and couldn't figure out how I'd end up there before him night after night. I did mention to him I thought I might be pregnant but coming after about six false alarms over the previous six months meant he didn't really believe me. "Oh yeah, I've heard that one before!"

I didn't want to take a pregnancy test for a few reasons. The bloody things were expensive for starters. I felt like it was akin to flushing my money down the toilet. Ten euros a go for two test sticks – the money wasn't long adding up. I had blown about thirty euros already with false alarms and wasn't going to waste another stick by peeing on it until I was sure. The main reason I didn't take a test though was probably because I was in a kind of denial myself. I knew if I confirmed I was pregnant I might think twice about my trip to the World Masters – and I really didn't want to do that. So in my twisted reasoning I decided that if I hadn't confirmed I was pregnant it would allow me to ride almost uninhibited – a bit crazy but it worked for me.

In terms of other symptoms in the first trimester I was lucky in that I didn't suffer any dramatic morning sickness. Many foods didn't really taste right though, and I did develop an aversion to some things. I developed a craving for acidic foods like grapefruits and orange juice – I just couldn't get enough of them. When I look back on it, this "slightly off" or odd feeling I had felt first in Croatia really lasted the whole of the first trimester. Some days it was worse than others. From talking to lots of girls, I think nearly everyone suffers from some sort of pregnancy symptoms in the first trimester. The reason this stage of pregnancy has the most dramatic symptoms is the body's physiology is undergoing such rapid changes it takes time for it to adapt.

This is probably the most likely reason a lot of people give up exercising in the first trimester. You could feel permanently nauseous or you might feel so tired you're not able for any strenuous activity at all. I frequently felt tired and unable to exercise which was a bit of a shock to me. However, since I was on a schedule heading for Manchester, not to mention paranoid about losing fitness, I was motivated to get out and do something most days. The funny thing was that even though I may not have remotely felt like going out for a run or to the gym, going for a long spin on the bike or doing a training session at the track, I had to admit that once I was out the door and had started exercising it not only gave me energy, but greatly improved my mood and general sense of wellbeing. I found that it was the only thing that would allow me to shrug off that odd edgy feeling that characterised my first trimester and gave me a feeling of normality for the rest of the day. The days I exercised were the days I felt best.

The motivation to get out there and get going was more than occasionally hard, but I'd encourage anyone to force themselves to make an effort to do something at this stage, even if they don't feel like it. As you will see I'm a big believer in listening to your body and letting that be the guide to what you do or don't do. But this is one case where the body need a little gentle encouragement or on some days even a good kick in the backside. Guaranteed, you will feel better afterwards. Of course if it's not happening for you after 15 minutes, you should go home again and give yourself a break. I think in all the time I was pregnant, even though I started countless exercise sessions feeling less than enthusiastic, I only had to pull the plug once or twice.

More importantly, I discovered from reading Dr Clapp's book there are very sound physiological reasons for getting out there and making the effort to exercise during the first trimester, especially if you want to continue with your exercise right through pregnancy. One of the effects of exercising at this early stage is that it greatly stimulates the early growth of the placenta and the extent of its blood supply. Clapp found that women who exercised strenuously during early pregnancy had much larger placentas with a greater blood supply then their sedentary counterparts. This adaptation increases the capacity of the placenta above normal, allowing the fetus to cope better with any stress, exercise induced or otherwise, in later pregnancy. Exercise during this early stage also enhances other facets of the maternal adaptations to pregnancy, such as improving the ability to dissipate extra heat through increased sweating and breathing. Basically, early benefits provide a margin of safety which allows women to train harder later in the pregnancy when they generally feel more able for it.

It was only when I started investigating the physiological changes the body is undergoing in this early stage that I discovered the reason I was so exhausted, not to mention the reason behind the frequent bathroom breaks. Pregnancy causes many dramatic changes in the body and as I mentioned previously these are mostly felt in the first trimester before the body adapts. Firstly, the heart and the circulatory system changes dramatically to accommodate the growth of the baby. These changes are responsible for many of the early symptoms of pregnancy, such as dizziness, nausea, overwhelming waves of fatigue, constipation, feeling bloated, frequent trips to the loo, etc. All these changes happen very early on.

Once the fertilized egg implants, a series of hormonal signals are triggered which cause a decrease in the peripheral resistance of the maternal blood vessels, literally overnight. This effectively means that there is a large increase in the volume of the woman's circulatory system, and suddenly not enough blood to fill it, basically it's like losing a pint or two of blood. As a result of this, the blood pressure falls, which can lead to feelings of nausea and dizziness. This change itself also leads to another effect. The body signals to the kidneys that there is not enough fluid in the circulatory system so the kidneys start to decrease the excretion of salt and water in an attempt to fill the newly expanded system again. Once this adaptation process is complete, both the blood volume and the cardiac output (amount of blood the heart pumps with each beat) have increased by a staggering 40%. The body adapts to these changes over time and usually it takes until the fourth month of pregnancy for most people feel normal again.

This increase in blood volume and flow has two other important effects. Firstly, the blood flow to the skin is greatly increased, raising skin temperature. This allows the pregnant woman to dissipate heat very efficiently and is also responsible for that pregnancy "glow". It also explains why you may frequently find yourself stripping off layers of clothing when everyone around you is wrapped up in their winter woollies. This adaptation is very useful during exercise as it allows greater dispersion of any surplus heat generated. This lets us to exercise, within reason, without putting the baby under any undue temperature stress. Secondly, the increase in blood flow is also marked in the kidneys, to increase filtration and removal of metabolic waste products, and is the reason behind those frequent trips to the loo, both day and night. This increased volume of urine can be very tiresome, especially when out running or cycling. As the pregnant uterus grows the "need-to-pee" effect is compounded by the pressure it places directly on the bladder.

There are interesting parallels between these circulatory adaptations to pregnancy and general adaptations to exercise the body makes in trained individuals. Like pregnancy, regular training also results in an increase in both blood volume and cardiac output. As mentioned earlier, regular training also increases the bodies capacity to dissipate body heat more efficiently form the skin surface, by effectively lowering the temperature required for the body to increase blood flow to the skin and initiate sweating. Another parallel that happens in the exercising individual is that the capacity of the circulatory system is increased, albeit in a slightly different way. Instead of a drop in peripheral resistance as happens with pregnancy, the blood systems' capacity increases due to increased vessel growth to the body tissues that need them, in order to ensure sufficient delivery of oxygen and nutrients to exercising muscles.

What does this mean? Basically the circulatory status of a normal pregnant woman at rest has many similarities with that of a trained non-pregnant person during exercise. Because of this, when a fit woman maintains her exercise regime during pregnancy, the cardiovascular adaptations from carrying a baby are superimposed on the preexisting adaptations to training, and the effects are additive. One study mentioned in Dr Clapp's book by a researcher called Pivarnik showed that the plasma volumes, red cell volumes and total blood volumes of regularly exercising women during pregnancy are at least 10-15% higher than their pregnant sedentary sisters. That's a big boost to the oxygen carrying system, enhancing the capacity for exercise.

One of the more common concerns I came across in discussions on exercise during pregnancy was the fact that heat stress could potentially have a teratogenic effect, or in simple terms cause malformations in the embryo. The interesting thing about this is there actually isn't any evidence that heat stress can cause these effects in humans, findings have been extrapolated from studies on rats. There is probably more of a reason to be concerned that extremely high temperatures could lead to abortion, as happens sometimes when the mother experiences an extremely high fever during illness. There may also be other factors related to the infectious agents at play here as well as the fever. But it is better to consider that extreme temperature stress may be risky until evidence comes to light to the contrary.

There are no reports to date in the literature of a woman losing a baby due to exercise induced heat-stress. In fact the body is actually in a good position to manage heat when in the pregnant state. The fact is the thermal adaptations from both pregnancy and training actually complement each other. This means that the risk of inducing a significant hike in body temperature due to exercise is extremely small, unless exercising to exhaustion, while under-hydrated or in extremely hot conditions. Not problems we here in Ireland have to deal with any time soon. In fact, being pregnant during the winter, I found the problem was staying warm on the bike as opposed to the opposite.

As it turns out there are many physiological changes that the body undergoes during pregnancy enabling the body to deal with exercise induced heat production (Modified from Dr Clapp's book):

1. The body's internal thermometer set point decreases
2. The blood flow increases to the skin to dissipate heat
3. The body's temperature that triggers sweating is lowered
4. Heat loss through breathing increases by 40-50%
5. The increased weight gain and blood volume buffer increases in heat production

I have to say I was relieved when I discovered the body has this suite of adaptations to spare the baby from heat stress. Being rather fond of the sauna after I finish a gym session, I wondered would it be safe to continue. There were warning signs on all saunas not use them when pregnant. Being me however I decided to do my own research into this. When I went about investigating whether it was safe I found some Finnish women continued to regularly use saunas right throughout their pregnancies. There was, however, a tendency towards shorter sessions, 10-15 minutes at a time. I decided I would continue as if I were Finnish too and frequently used the sauna. There is one legitimate reason to be careful of the sauna when in the early stages of pregnancy in particular. If you have very low blood pressure, which can frequently happen in the first trimester, the blood vessels dilate as you heat up. Your blood pressure can fall further and you may be at risk of passing out, so caution is required. On the subject of the hot tub, I had initially thought you weren't supposed to use them due to risk of infection, but I subsequently discovered it's a whole lot easier to overheat in one than in a sauna, due to the fact that water is a far more effective heat conductor then air. Having said that, as the temperature is quite low in the one in my gym I did use it occasionally.

All in all during the first trimester I pretty much continued my exercise and racing as normal. Partly because I was in denial but more so because, from what I had learned, I felt it was acceptable to do so. I felt that exercising through my pregnancy was going to be a positive thing, both for me, my pregnancy and the baby. My own knowledge and gut instinct told me this, but my feelings were reinforced by Dr Clapp's research, the Professor's advice and all the other scientific papers I had read on the topic which gave me the confidence to go on. Looking back at my training diary I was doing anything between five to eight hours exercise a week during the first trimester. Most of the hours training I was doing was time spent on the bike. The time consisted of one long spin of maybe two to three hours, than the rest of the time was made of specific sessions on the track with very targeted technical drills. Most of the training was of moderate intensity and aerobic. In terms of higher intensity work I was probably doing about an hour of that a week during the races I was participating in at this time, in both the track league and the national and regional track championships and cyclo-cross near the end of the first trimester, which I will talk a bit more about later. I was also going swimming and jogging occasionally in spite of Hugh's advice about it slowing my leg speed. During this time the fact that I had signed up for the Masters in October was what motivated me to keep training and keep things ticking over.

How did I feel during all this, training as normal? Some days I felt great, other days a bit sluggish. It was very variable. I wore a heart rate monitor for a while at the start, but my heart rate was all over the place no matter what I was doing, so deciding it was of limited use, I ditched it early on. I had also read in a few different studies that heart rate could be highly variable and wasn't a particularly good guide to use, and that the Borg scale of perceived exertion was probably a better measure of what level to exercise at during pregnancy. When I look back, I don't think that being pregnant really had a massive impact on my performance in the first trimester, either when training or racing. Yes I felt more out of breath on occasion but my times weren't vastly different to before the pregnancy. Looking back at the Masters I definitely think I could have achieved a better overall placing in the bunch race I did but it was more the psychological side of things that held me back. Being seven or eight weeks pregnant I didn't want to be totally irresponsible and fall off while taking chances going for the sprint finish.

Once I got over the Masters (and more to the point survived it and felt good) I had such a taste for competing I didn't want to stop. I felt fine when racing so decided to go on for a while at least. Over the next few months I participated in the Dublin cyclocross league, or the "Supercross Cup" as it's commonly known. I had always been intrigued by this alternative cycling discipline – a sort of a cross over between road and mountain biking, for hardcore deranged people who didn't mind getting covered in mud and freezing their asses off during winter, as the season runs in the coldest months, from October to January. The races take place in a number of different public parks around Dublin and are short and intense, usually less than an hour. A race consists of a number of laps each up to two kilometers in length on a technical course. There is usually a range of obstacles to negotiate, steep sharp corners, steps, jump boards, short hills, roots, grass and mud. And more mud. It depended on the weather, but there could be lots of it. The more the better it seemed. And there was usually no shortage of it with all the rain we get in Ireland during those autumn and winter months.

Cyclocross racing is technical and fast, carried out on what are basically road bikes with grippy knobbly tyres and slightly different brakes. Due to the nature of the racing there are not to many girls involved, in fact it's even less popular with women than mountain biking. I think the most girls in any one race during the series that year was six. Because of the small numbers you have to race with the guys which means the pace is pretty fast. The starts are pretty hairy and there can be a lot of elbows and wheels clashing and then if you're lucky enough to stay upright its ride at your limit until the finish. The fastest people in a race will nearly always lap the slowest at least once. Once you're lapped, its race over, sometimes a blessing in disguise.

During the season there were practice sessions once a week in a park on the outskirts of Dublin. The first time I attended one of these I thought it was a bit crazy. I thought I must be mad to be participating in this, and nearly went home. The sessions took place weather regardless, in the coldest and wettest of conditions, by the lights of the nearby motorway, the M50. The park where the sessions took place was adjacent to the motorway and there was barely enough light from the massive sodium lamps to see where you were going in the park, in fact just about enough illumination to stop you riding into the back of someone else, once your eyes adjusted. There was of course the option of riding with bike lights but there was an unwritten rule against this, and silent disapproval or anyone who did. I understood why after I was blinded by some guy riding towards me with an extremely bright headlamp. The course we trained on was marked out each evening by Robin Seymour, multiple Irish Cyclocross champion, and his clubmates, Team WORC using small white plastic poles with flashing red rear bike lights on top. We would do lap efforts and work on skills and just when we were getting tired and thinking this session must be nearly over Robin would say "Now it's time to race!" Robin was a seriously talented rider, having competed for Ireland at Olympic level in mountain biking and even though in his 40s was still an amazing athlete. He had no problem beating all the young up and coming talented riders in most of the races. So race we would do. These nights of training would toughen anyone up. I remember one particular evening during training I skidded on my bike when cornering and fell off. A split second of panic in midair as I thought "Oh God, I'm pregnant!" Then a nice soft thunk as my backside and right thigh slid to the ground. "I hardly felt that!" I thought. I reckoned the nature of the falls during cyclocross weren't too bad, and there wasn't any risk of abdominal trauma which gave me the peace of mind to continue.

For added training benefit I cycled all the way from home to the park and back, which added a good hour and a half riding to the hour long session itself. I shiver thinking back on those sessions now as I write. I remember distinctly acknowledging one particularly bitter windy dark November night my madness, shivering my way home, looking wistfully through windows of warm sitting rooms as I cycled past and couldn't warm up. Yes it was hard going, but also exhilarating, which made it worthwhile.

In 2011, I raced most of the series that made up the Supercross Cup in the cyclocross league. After winning my first race, I felt I had to continue. If I competed in four of five of the races and came out on top I could win the overall ladies prize. As it turned out I was first girl in all the races I did. I was nearly four months pregnant competing in the final race and was kind of glad that was the end of it. I had noticed over the previous few weeks that though I was training consistently and my cyclocross skills were improving, I seemed to be getting slightly slower in comparison to the guys I was racing against. I think that from the three month mark on I was definitely slowing, even though putting in what I felt was the same effort. It was a natural end to my racing season. I regrettably opted to skip the cyclocross nationals in January 2012 as at that stage I would be five months and I felt it would be pushing my limits of risk. By the time the Nationals rolled around I knew it would have been a bad idea. Sense eventually prevailed and I hung up my cleats.

SECOND TRIMESTER – COMING CLEAN

The second trimester was marked by my coming clean, or admitting I was pregnant, to a number of people, including myself. It started at the end of October with my taking a pregnancy test – I was so pregnant the line was in the box before I even removed the stick from my stream of pee. Not that I needed it to tell me what I already knew but there was a certain shock in confirming it to myself. I really had to face up to it now. I talked to Cormac about it that night. I took a deep breath and dropped the bombshell. "I'm definitely pregnant", I told him over dinner. "Get out – you are not! Here we go again, another false alarm!" He really didn't believe me. I showed him the stick with the incriminating line (which was still there thankfully). Only then did he actually accept it and believe what I was telling him. "Why do you think I've been crawling into my bed at nine or ten every night and getting up to pee at frequent intervals? Or not drinking tea or eating as normal? Or consuming litres of orange juice? Did you not notice there was something up with me?" "Not really but I suppose now that you mention it.", he mulled it over. "Well that's great news! What's for dessert?" My God, I could hardly believe his reaction. This thing had been constantly playing in the back of my mind for the last three months and he wasn't even tuning in. "Such is the lot of the one having to carry the baby around", I sighed. It was probably going to take a while for it to sink in I reckoned so let him off the hook.

When it came to my training, even though I felt I was operating within comfortable limits, I suppose I had been going along on a bit of a wing and a prayer but I felt I really needed to find out a bit more about what was possible to do and put some structure to what I was doing. I felt like I was floundering around a bit. I really wanted to talk first-hand to someone who had been in the same situation, but didn't think the likes of Sonia O'Sullivan would appreciate my cold-calling her. I also had something big hanging over me – I had to tell my coach, Hugh. That was the one piece of advice Cormac gave me straight away – I had to tell him as it wasn't fair not to. I had never had a coach until two months before and I was really benefitting from it. Hugh was super and was getting the best out of me at every juncture, considering my lack of experience. I really didn't want to lose his input. It was so nice for a change to have someone helping me achieve my best in a sport. I had never had a coach before. I was terrified he would not take me seriously, though, once he found out about the pregnancy. I knew I wanted to keep training as much as I could and I realised I wanted his help, but most of all his support. I knew I had to keep training as best I could were I to have any chance at fulfilling my dream returning to the Masters in a competitive state the following October. Most of all I knew I needed to keep training for my own sanity and felt it would help preserve my identity. I knew this would be easier if I had someone with some objectivity to support me and keep me motivated throughout and Hugh could do this. I had to consider the possibility that Hugh would refuse to continue coaching me at all because of my condition, as would be his right. I knew it was going to be a shock when I told him and felt bad for not telling him sooner. About a week after I told Cormac and my parents I attended a talk on winter training one night at the club house. Afterwards Hugh gave me a lift home as I was stranded having to leave my bike in for some maintenance. I knew this was my opportunity. As we pulled up outside the house I just blurted it out. "I've something to tell you. I'm pregnant. But I want to keep training right through. It's OK. I've looked into it. It's safe and lots of athletes do it." The look of shock on his face was something to behold. He really didn't see it coming at all. He didn't say much. I could see he was well outside his comfort zone. After a few moments silence as it sunk in he asked me how far along was I. "Three months! You're joking! This is a lot to take in. Just leave it with me. I'll have a think about it and we can talk tomorrow." As he drove off still in shock I wondered would he come back and tell me he didn't want to coach me anymore. When I asked him months later how he felt at that moment he explained what had been going on in his head. His initial reaction was shock as he hadn't seen it coming. He told me that this was because during training sessions I always appeared to be very focused on what I were planning to do on the track the following year and that was always part of our conversations. Although I told him I was pregnant at an early stage he admitted he felt a bit ambushed, having been coaching me for all those weeks and not knowing I had a passenger on board. With absolutely no experience in coaching pregnant women and no desire to do so before I came along, he was hesitant to take on the responsibility. Before this Hugh said he had heard that many athletes came back post birth stronger but had no idea of what they would have been capable of during their term. He knew that some women maintained fitness throughout the pregnancy but he didn't know or understand the limiting factors. After he reflected on it for a few days he told me the idea grew on him and he was actually quite excited about it all as he saw it as a challenge and a chance to learn something new. Finally, which was very nice of him, he admitted that he couldn't desert me, although had he not been training me already he admits he would have probably refused! But he knew how important it was to me to keep going and that I desperately needed someone's help and support to do it. How could he say no?

After he told me all this I thought his opinions might make some interesting reading in the book and give a different angle on things. He put a piece together around the end of the second trimester for me and it went as follows:

"Even though I mightn't have gone out of my way to take it on, I found coaching a pregnant female rider has been a very positive experience. As a coach it is essential that you are told as early as possible so you can plan the workload accordingly and know that you are working on a long-term plan, with some goals having to be put on the long finger. This was my first experience of dealing with this situation and it was a steep and interesting learning curve .

When Susie told me she wanted to keep training and would like me to keep coaching her through her pregnancy, I was very aware that I lacked the particular experience needed and it did take a bit of time to work it all out. Even though Susie expressed a fear that I might shy away from the challenge and not take her seriously, I assured her that I wouldn't desert her since I had already agreed to help her. It was just that I wasn't really sure exactly how.

After digesting the news for 24 hours I came up with a very cunning plan - I would ask for help! Luckily, I knew a top level national rider who had recently given birth, maintained her fitness throughout and made a successful return to international standards. I asked if she would meet with my rider and I, to work through some possibilities and she agreed to help. She was also a medical doctor and understood all that we needed to know, from the perspective of a medical and sporting background. We three met and Susie had a list of questions and I sat back and listened intently. I wanted to understand what the possibilities and limits would be at the various stages and I knew I had a duty of care to both mother and baby so I needed to have all this very clear in my head. This turned out to be one of my better ideas, and I had a whole lot more knowledge about training and pregnancy in general on the way out! I realised afterwards we would need to select appropriate training methods and modify them as the pregnancy progressed, some drills and exercises would be more suitable than others at each stage. I also realised that we were not working for peak fitness as we would be coming up to a major competition , but the most important thing was to maintain a certain level of fitness and work to maintain and develop strength and flexibility and probably even more importantly to use it as a time to improve technique. Mental imagery and focus on long term goals were also important during this period to keep Susie sane in the realization she would come back even stronger. My job as a coach was to ensure she saw it as a positive time for her athletic development. I realised it was also essential that at no point pressure be applied for any workload to be undertaken and that the athlete is assured that letting go is OK if that is the right thing at the time. Luckily, Susie was from a medical background as such she was familiar with how to research various articles and papers, which helped us make informed decisions as to what was possible and worked best for mother and baby.

As a coach you too are responsible for safety of both mother and child so once armed with all relevant parameters you set the limits. Safety is all about minimising and controlling any risk and this is done by attention to detail. Many of these things I was already doing as we trained together, but I wanted to ensure that when she was training with anyone else that these standards were understood and adhered to so I devised a set of rules for safe cycling.

It is a unique thing working with a pregnant athlete. You have to help them be well placed for their comeback but also recognise that their view on how important all those goals were might very well change once they give birth. Priorities completely change with the arrival of a child. However, in my experience, women who pursue their sporting goals after giving birth tend to be supercharged. I have learned much from this experience and it has greatly improved me as a coach. It has also given me even more respect for Susie as an athlete and as a person and am very happy to continue the journey should she choose to."

Good old Hugh, of course he wasn't going to let me down. As he mentions in his piece he did the one thing I knew would be most helpful for me. He put me in touch with someone who had been there. He contacted a friend of his, a girl who was at the time was training with the Irish ladies Team Pursuit squad. At the time these girls were trying to qualify for London 2012. This girl had just had a baby the previous Christmas. I had heard on the grapevine that she was back training very quickly after giving birth and had seen her at the Irish Track Nationals where she had been on the podium a few times, with her baby in tow.

She responded immediately with enthusiasm when Hugh asked for a meeting and we were around in her house the following evening for tea and a chat. It was so good to talk to her. Such a positive girl and she was a great help to me. She told me how she stayed in the gym right up till the end lifting weights (nothing too heavy, but still doing squats and the like). She told me how she had stayed competing in the first few months doing time trials mostly (which made me feel less reckless for doing the Masters and currently competing in the cyclocross). She told me how she stayed on the bike till she was 30 weeks pregnant. I asked her why she used this as her cut off and her reasoning was that while your bump is relatively small the baby is pretty well protected but when you start to get bigger, with more out front of course, the baby is more vulnerable to trauma should you be unlucky enough to fall. That made sense. She advised me to use the cross trainer and rowing machines in the gym as they are great especially when your bump gets bigger. She also told me she was back training ten days after giving birth and was so ecstatic to be back in the gym she was nearly falling off the machines! This was all good stuff, music to my ears. This girl clearly hadn't lost her desire to exercise or competitive edge which I found very heartening. I bounced out of there with a new lease of life, totally thrilled to have met her. Hugh had much more confidence to go on too. He said, "First thing I'll do is make a plan for safe cycling. We need to set some rules in place to optimise your safety. There's no reason why you can't continue on the bike for a long time yet as long as we take the right approach". At that Hugh went off and devised a set of rules to optimise my safety when I was on the bike and emailed me the following day:

Hi Susie,

I will list definite nos, limiters and some safety elements I want you to follow.

Nos
(1) No more group rides - too many variables and we can't put your safety in other people's hands. Also you need to be going at your pace (more about that later).
(2) No rev outs (these are drills where you practice high leg speed) - This counts for rollers too. No worries about backing off as all this training is neuromuscular and that will come back very quickly.
(3) Slightest hint of frost - no ride at all.
(4) Wet roads - no ride.
(5) No climbing serious hills and especially no fast descents.

Limiters
(1) Company - You can ride on the road for as long as you feel able but with one other rider only and their job is to look after you.
(2) Pace - Main thing about this is just to match whatever pace you set. This is a skill that appears to be easy but one that not everyone can do. Main thing is never to stick your wheel in front of the person you are pacing but also keep it steady - no surges.
(3) Rider position - you have to be always on the inside but the other thing would be that if road narrows then other rider rides behind (a bike length distance behind your rear wheel) and slightly to the right of you rear wheel (about a foot). This gives you extra clearance from overtaking cars and more importantly allows you a clear view of the road that getting shelter from the wind. Also, if you are in front for these short periods you are still setting your pace and no danger of hitting a rear wheel. For your part - no looking around!! There is much more protection given to you by rider riding behind.
(4) Train within comfortable limits - Either use your heart rate monitor - 70% Max. This means max - not train at! Or gauge your effort using the Borg Scale of perceived exertion.
(5) Nutrition and hydration - more than ever you need to have a drink and food with you especially on longer spins and make sure you eat and drink frequently - as you can't afford to have any lapses in concentration due to lack of energy. Means to fix a puncture would be good too.
(6) Rides on quiet roads with very little traffic are optimal. If necessary

you can drive and meet someone on the outskirts of the city.

Options
(1) Firstly you don't have to train at all - this is your choice and I trust you to listen to your body. I firmly believe you will achieve all you would wish for no matter which path you take.
(2) The aerobic side of things can be maintained in other ways like turbo instead of rollers, swimming, cross trainer, etc.
(3) Cut back - lower weights, less time on rollers (Max 45 min), train less times per week , etc.

In short, don't be afraid to let go as we all know you will come back stronger. Also, remember that easy spins are the friend of the sprinter and think long-term which we were doing anyway. Good to work with you as apart from helping you to develop your true potential, my own form has improved significantly. I feel as a coach the key to keeping ones enthusiasm is to do as much training with your riders as possible and it has been a useful insight into how to work with pregnant athletes - although this is definitely a once-off. Would not have chosen it but as I was already working with you, I wouldn't refuse to help. As a coach too it is gratifying to work with someone who I believe in and who responds so well to training so anything I can do for you - more than happy to do.

Regards, Hugh

As I mulled this over I thought it was generally pretty sound advice. Hugh was so supportive – something that really gave me added confidence to go on and not to ditch the bike. That was really important to me. Of course I was a little wary of continuing cycling but by putting all Hugh's rules into action I felt a lot more comfortable. I was a bit sad at not going on any more group rides with Sundrive as I had been really enjoying the camaraderie and the social aspects of the spins. However, I had to acknowledge the previous Sunday I had been feeling the pressure a bit physically at the start of the spin. It was probably about time to pull the plug. I was also starting to tune into how it was a bit more dangerous to ride in a group after a few people had crashed on a slippery section of road during the previous week's spin and didn't want to be in the middle of that either. So with a little regret I waved goodbye to my Sundrive teammates.

I continued to go out on long road spins but now only with one other person, as suggested by my new guidelines. My performance on the bike during these spins in the second trimester was quite variable. Some days it could take me about an hour or so to really get going, I tended to be pretty sluggish at the start of a spin. Hugh frequently accompanied me during this time. Every second week he had a day off and as I was working three days a week I would also frequently be off so it suited both of us. Hugh had noticed that my pace was slower than normal but was happy to roll along and he commented on how much stronger I nearly always was on the return leg.

We usually covered about 80km on these long spins. Despite all the advice to the contrary that the duration of exercise sessions should be reduced during pregnancy, I found being out on the bike for three or four hours was no problem, as long as the pace was maintained at a level I felt comfortable at on the day. I would also insist on a mandatory coffee stop in the middle of these spins regardless of who was with me, and always made a point of eating a massive scone with my coffee at these stopovers. This extra sustenance would put me in great form to power back home. I really enjoyed those cups of coffee too. I had gone off tea right from the start of pregnancy but still loved that one cup of coffee mid-morning. All in all including the coffee stops I would usually be out for about four hours. My pace would usually average out at about 25kph, probably 22-23kph on the way out and 26-27kph on the way home, all fuelled up on scones and coffee. I never pushed the pace on a spin; it was just about whatever I felt comfortable doing on the day. I never worried about how long I was out either, reasoning as long as I stayed well hydrated and ate plenty before and during the spin, I would be fine, which I was. I had also decided that I would listen to Hugh's friend's advice and keep going on the road until I was 30 weeks pregnant, as long as my bump didn't get too big before then. This and following the rules Hugh set out, made me feel pretty safe and confident I was making the right decision.

Around this time my husband and I went to visit a friend in Barcelona. He was married to a Spanish girl, Maria, who was also pregnant and due the same time as I. She was horrified to hear I was doing such long cycles and didn't think it was safe and started to lecture me about it. The ironic thing was she herself was cycling to work every day on busy Barcelona streets. "But it's only 15 minutes each way", she protested.

"Yes," I said, "15 minutes in which you've a fair chance of being knocked off your bike by a crazy Spanish driver in rush hour." Safety is definitely relative.

I did have one pregnancy complication at this time and it was really affecting my cycling, severe heartburn. It was particularly bad in the second trimester and continued to the end without relief. Whatever it was about the position on the bike, the heartburn was worse when I was in the saddle. I tried all sorts of natural remedies, avoided certain foods, ate others, but nothing worked. I eventually gave into the over the counter drugs. I found Gaviscon fantastic. For ages I was hefting around a 300ml glass bottle of it in the back of my cycling jersey and would get very odd looks from people as I surreptitiously pulled it from my pocket for a swig, while they were munching bananas and energy bars. Later on I discovered Gaviscon came in these fantastic (albeit, outrageously overpriced) single sachets, which were much more portable. For the belt and braces approach I always threw a good heaped spoon of Andrews liver salts into my water bottle. I'm not joking when I say the heartburn was bad though. I went out on a spin once without my remedies and had to turn for home after twenty minutes of agony.

There was still one person left I had to come clean with. With husband and coach out of the way, the last man standing was my boss at work. This was the one I had been dreading. A number of years ago I remembered reading about a British MEP, Godfrey Bloom, who was trying to overturn maternity leave rights in the European parliament. He became famous for his words which were quoted in the Guardian newspaper: "No self-respecting small businessman with a brain in the right place would ever employ a woman of child-bearing age." Even though his comment was indeed highly sexist and inflammatory, it was also true. I hated the way there was no equality when it came to who minded the baby in Ireland, and most of southern Europe for that matter. As far as I was concerned, only the Scandinavians had it right. I had worked in Norway the previous year and learned that the father and mother could split the paid leave to mind the baby as it suited them. What's more the father *had* to take 9 weeks of this paid leave or the couple lost it completely. We are so backward in Ireland I felt, mostly courtesy of the outdated Irish constitution, which basically states "a woman's place is in the home". I read a bit about parental equality in relation to maternity leave around this time as had the notion it might be nice for Cormac to take some of the leave, allowing me to go back to work a bit earlier, but realised very quickly that there was no chance of this happening. There had been legal challenges in Europe which had failed where fathers had wanted to take the leave instead of mothers. So I had to face the music and tell my boss the good news, that I would be gone for the whole summer and autumn, the busiest time of the year for we fish vets.

At the time I worked at a veterinary practice based in Galway in the west of Ireland but my job took me all over the country. It was just me and Hamish, my boss. Most of our work was on salmon farms located off the Irish west coast, usually in remote and beautiful locations. We also visited freshwater farms which were inland, as this is where salmon start their life and grow to a certain size before they are ready to go to sea. I loved my job. I had previously worked as both a large and companion animal vet, but found fish medicine so interesting, once I got a taste of it there was no going back. There were always new challenges for us to help the industry stay ahead of. No more than any type of farming, there were disease challenges and health strategies to be worked out. Every site was different and had its own issues. Fish-farming has become a hugely important industry with the decline of global wild fisheries around the world. I liked working with the industry in Ireland as we were taking advantage of our "clean green little island in the middle of nowhere" image and the majority of sites were producing high quality organic salmon. Most Irish people don't realise the quality of the salmon produced in Ireland as most of it is exported to countries like Germany and France – they pay a premium price for it and in fact can't get enough of it in Europe.

People are always asking me what a fish vet does. A normal day's work for me might first involve driving a few hours to a site, as most fish farms are in remote coastal locations. Then I would be transported by boat with my gear out to the pens where the fish are held to examine the salmon. During routine health checks I would capture and anesthetise a few fish from different pens and all looking well return them after examination. If I were visiting a site in response to a disease outbreak, I'd sample what we call moribund (sick) fish for examination and euthanize a few for histology. Histology sampling involves taking small pieces of all the different organs and preserving them in formalin.

The tissues are then processed in a specialist lab, slides made and sent back to us so we can screen them under the microscope. This enables us to hopefully figure out what is going on with the fish as we can have a detailed look at all the internal organs microscopically. I might also do some bacteriology or take blood samples for virology if I think it's indicated. One of the things I loved about my job was the fact that we did everything – from the pen-side examination and sampling of the fish, to reading the slides and interpreting the other clinical results. You could see the case through from start to finish, and that doesn't really happen in any other type of veterinary medicine. To keep us going in addition to the clinical visits we are usually also involved in some type of research project. Gills were the flavour of the month around the time I was pregnant as they had become an important disease issue in the industry. I had just handed in my PhD at the end of October on the bacteria that cause gill disease in Atlantic salmon, work which I had presented at that conference in Croatia when I realised I was pregnant. Finally, Hamish and I frequently ran training workshops on all aspects of fish health and welfare.

I was really worried about how my boss would react when I told him the news. I had managed to keep my pregnancy under wraps for five months, but knew when I went back after Christmas I was getting to the point where I would have to come clean. The job was occasionally very physical, and could involve long hours, rough seas, inclement weather, jumping on and off boats, pulling nets and hefting large salmon around. I was doing fine workwise and didn't find the pregnancy was affecting my ability to work at all but didn't know how he would view it. The only thing I had noticed was I occasionally felt mildly nauseous when out on a rolling swell, something that had never happened before I was pregnant. The day I came back to work after the holidays in January, we were wrapping up our usual catch up meeting when he asked was there anything else we needed to discuss. "I've something to tell you," I blurted out, "I'm bloody pregnant!" He looked so shocked, his face was a study. I don't know what he thought I was going to say, but in fairness to him he recovered fairly quickly. "That's great news! Congratulations. How far along are you?" "5 months I replied". "What??" "Did you not notice, or did you just think I was getting fat?" I joked. "So when are you due?" he asked, shocked for a second time, and trying to process the news, "We'll have to try getting a replacement for you." "There's no rush, I'm absolutely fine to do my job and want to work right up till the end," I informed him. "Right so, we'll see", he replied as he mulled it over, "Just let me know what you're able for and we'll play it by ear." By the following week I discovered he had told some of the fish farmers. One of the girls working on a site had sent me a mail congratulating me. "Why did you tell them," I wailed, "now they will be treating me with kid gloves, and I'm grand. I'm fitter and stronger than most non-pregnant women!" "Yes Susie that may be true but they need to know. What if you're out at sea and go into labour?" "I won't though", I said, "My mum was late with all of us so I'd say I'll be the same!" He didn't look too convinced. "And I was doing so well hiding it – I'd say I could go all the way to the end with these oilskins covering my bump and no one would have noticed!"

But the cat was out of the bag. Thankfully by and large I wasn't treated any differently. He had only told a few key people so most of the staff on the farms didn't know, and I was doing a great job hiding my small bump in my oilskins. We started to look for someone to replace me and it wasn't easy. That's the problem with such a specialised job. I tried to convince some new vet graduates to give it a go but despite my hard sell and encouragement to try something different, they were still in four-legged furry mode. All most people want to do when they leave vet college is work with four legged animals and encouraging them to think laterally at this point was a waste of time. I knew as I had been there to.

With the problems we were encountering finding a replacement for me I was feeling a bit guilty leaving Hamish in the lurch, especially at the start of the busy season for us. I promised him I would be back as soon as I could and we would aim roughly for October, when the baby would be four to five months old. Finally, we found an American girl who had studied in Scotland with an interest in fish who was prepared to give it a shot. "I'm sure she will be grand", I reassured Hamish, when he expressed concern that she would find the job too challenging. We knew it would be a bit of a mission to sort her with a visa but Hamish reckoned he could do it. I was able to relax after that and breathe a sigh of relief.

Meanwhile Hugh had been busy coming up with a plan for how I could modify my training to optimise my time since I probably wouldn't be able to effectively maintain things like high intensity efforts much longer. He decided that since we couldn't focus on optimising sprinting ability or lactate threshold, it was a good opportunity to focus on cadence, a factor that is just as important for cycling performance, particularly on the track. Cadence, or leg speed, is very important for all track disciplines, much more so than for road cycling. Some people are naturally better than others at working at high cadence, but it can also be trained and improved greatly with practice. It was a perfect time to put some energy into developing this aspect of my cycling, and I was delighted to have something concrete to work on. It felt like the limits were being lifted. Optimum cadence for road cycling is probably around 90rpm (cadence is measured in revolutions per minute or "rpm", basically the number of times your pedals make a full revolution in one minute) but for different track disciplines the figures are much higher. The reason for this is that track bikes only have one gear, which is also the gear you have to start in so it needs to be easy enough to get going, therefore will require a lot of spinning to sustain higher speeds once you get going. Just to illustrate, cadences requirements for various track disciplines would be as follows:

Typical Cadences
-   Bunch race like a Scratch Race: 100rpm (duration approx 15 -30 minutes)
-   500m Time Trial: 125 rpm (duration approx 40 seconds)
-   Pursuit: 110-120 rpm (duration depends on distance, 2-4 minutes)
-   Flying 200: 145 – 160 rpm (duration approximately 12-15 seconds)

Getting your legs to these speeds without bouncing all over the place in the saddle is a skill that takes a lot of practice. Of course fitness plays a part too, but you have to train your nervous system and your muscles to pedal at this speed, and the shorter the interval the less your fitness helps to get your leg speed up to target. Most track riders work on leg speed and strength at different times in their training programmes and then marry the two later on. So you can generally practice and perfect these cadences using much lower gears then you would use in competition, and then ride the bigger gears once your legs have learned how to spin efficiently at the higher rpms. All round it was a great thing for me to focus on for a few months. I was able to work on cadence out on road spins, on a stationary trainer and in the gym. When I was out on road spins I dropped my gear to one below where I was comfortable, forcing me to spin my legs a bit more than normal. Around this time I also decided to purchase a form of stationary bike trainer. Instead of the more common turbo-trainer which most cyclists would use (a turbo-trainer consists of a frame, a clamp to hold the bicycle securely, a roller that presses up against the rear wheel, and a mechanism that provides resistance when the pedals are turned), I opted for a set of "rollers", a stationary trainer commonly used by track riders. With rollers, you have to balance on the bike when riding, as the bike just sits on top of three drums which spin when you pedal. The drums rotate in the opposite direction to your wheels, creating inertia and preventing the bike moving forward. Rollers force you to balance at all times since the bike's not locked in like on a turbo-trainer and this really helps to develop cycling-specific core strength. By practicing riding in a doorway for a few weeks I eventually got to grips with them and found them great. The rollers really helped smooth out my pedalling style which helped improve my cadence at the higher leg speeds. There is no room for bouncing in the saddle on rollers - you end up with a very sore backside very quickly if you don't learn how to ride smoothly.

In the gym, I frequently practiced another cadence drill which Hugh had devised for me, along with giving me the following important advice. "If you're using stationary bikes you must firstly set up saddle height correctly and take note of the setting. And don't even bother doing these workouts if the bike doesn't have toe-straps. Make sure you set these so that your foot is semi-wedged into a position with the ball of your foot over the pedal. Set the resistance pretty low. Level two or three is fine. This is about working on the neuromuscular system rather than the cardiovascular. It won't send your heart rate too high either. It's all about improving the cadence!" The workout was as follows:

0-8 min gradually increase cadence to be spinning about 100 rpm
@ 8 min spin at 120 rpm for 30 sec. Then easy spinning back down about 100 again.
@ 10 min spin at 130 rpm for 30 sec. Easy spinning (100 – 120 rpm).
@ 12 min spin at 140 rpm for 30 sec. Easy spinning (100 – 120 rpm).
@ 14 min spin at 150 rpm for 30 sec. Easy spinning (100 – 120 rpm).
@ 16 min spin at 160 rpm for 30 sec. Easy spinning (100 – 120 rpm).
@ 18 min spin at 170 rpm for 30 sec. Easy spinning (100 – 120 rpm).
@ 20 min spin at 180 rpm for 30 sec. Easy spinning (100 – 120 rpm).
@ 24 min make a 10 second burst to hit the highest cadence you can. Repeat this every two minutes three times.
@ 30 min easy spinning for 5 mins to warm down.

I did this session once or twice a week, depending on what else I managed to squeeze in and found it really helpful. I started to notice a difference in my pedalling after a few weeks. The other benefit of a session like this of course is it's done in a gym. This is great when it's dark, cold and wet outside. Also it's safe – to my knowledge no one has yet been run over while on a gym bike. Finally a session such as the one above is ideal in terms of keeping things interesting. I would die from boredom if someone told me to get up on a stationary bike for five let alone 35 minutes. But with this session half an hour has gone by before you feel it. Because this wasn't so hard on the legs, being done at a relatively low resistance, it was ideal to do before a weights session, and doubled up as a really good warm up.

That brings me onto the topic of lifting weights. Going against popular advice again, even though I hadn't ever really lifted too much before I was pregnant, I got into resistance training properly for the first time during my pregnancy. No matter what the trimester, I found it a great way to work out. I had thought doing weights was boring, probably a reflection of my general aversion to the gym before pregnancy, but enjoyed lifting once I settled into it at all and found it gave me a real sense of achievement. One of the things people say when I tell them I did a lot of weights when I was pregnant is "Oh that was OK for you, you were used to it". Quite the contrary in fact. I used to do the following when I went to the gym with a bit of variation depending on the availability of weights and machines and how I felt:

- Squats using the Olympic bar – I started just with the bar in the first trimester and worked my way up to 60 – 70kg, always lifting within my ability, never putting myself under too much pressure. I wanted to lift more on occasion and felt up for it but Hugh put the foot down and made me stop at 70. Because I was keeping the weight "light" I did high reps – usually three sets of 12-15 squats.
- Leg press – I used to do three sets of these (12-15 reps) with anything from 50 - 80 kg, depending on how I felt on the day.
- Bench press – I just used the un-weighted Olympic bar for this. When pregnant, you're not supposed to lie flat on your back when doing weights, as some women can get what's called "supine hypotension" – basically very low blood pressure. To

avoid this I always did bench presses with the bench at a 30-45 degree angle, usually three sets of 10 reps.

- Upward Row – I did this with about 20kg, three sets of 10 reps.
- Lat Pull-downs – I did these with about 25 - 30kg, three sets of 10 reps.

Every session without fail I also did at least 6-10 minutes of core work. In retrospect, I believe this was absolutely crucial to my recovery post-partum. Regular crunches should be avoided as they can put too much pressure on your *linea alba*, the connective tissue at the centre of your abs. Therefore I concentrated on planks as my main core exercise. I used to do three sets which lasted two minutes each: Front plank x 30 seconds, side plank left X 30s, side plank right X 30s then back to centre plank for the final 30 seconds. Then take a break. The other core exercise I did was side-to-sides with a 3kg medicine ball. You basically balance on your bum and hold the ball in both hands. Then you touch the ball to the ground beside you, alternating between your left and right sides. Do this for one minute then rest and repeat.

In summary, I found the upper body weights quite easy and my ability was not greatly affected by the pregnancy. I deliberately decided not to push too hard though as I didn't see the need and also didn't want to risk injury. The legs were a bit more challenging as they require more core involvement. The core work was challenging but I worked well within my comfort zone and it helped me keep the squats and leg press going. Hugh suggested that I do the combined cadence drill and weights session twice a week saying, "The bottom line is the priority for the moment is to maintain some strength but more than anything improve your cadence. It is not too taxing if done right. I know you always want to push it but we will have to claw back some of the adrenalin junkie in you and trust me that restraint will help here." He knew me so well. I needed the advice not to be afraid to let some things go as time went on.

That was one of the great things about Hugh. He gave me worthwhile tasks to focus on, but also organised other stuff for me to do as time went on to keep me motivated and ticking over. He made me understand there is so much more to training for something then just the physical elements. One example of this came in January 2012 when I was five months pregnant. He organised a special visit for me as a treat to keep me motivated – we went to get a proper bike-fit with Frank O'Connor out in Ritches bike shop in Swords in Dublin. Frank is a lovely guy, a super bike mechanic and his number one skill is fitting people properly on their bikes. He has fitted hundreds of people, everyone from professional cyclists to complete rookies. And I'm talking about doing it properly, not just measuring your inseam as they do in most bike shops! He takes loads of measurements and uses video analysis, lasers, funny bendy rulers and the like. He perfects everything from the position of your arms to the angle of your foot. I had always wanted to get a proper bike fit done as I knew it was important and bound to make a difference, especially on the track where every second counts. At this point, even though I was nearly five months pregnant, I asked Hugh not to tell Frank about my condition. I knew I could get away with it as I still wasn't really showing and with the help of a slightly baggy sweatshirt I'd look normal. The reason I didn't want him to know was that I was afraid he wouldn't take me seriously and that he would think I was wasting his time. Hugh understood and said he would say nothing. In retrospect once I got to know him, I know Frank wouldn't have even blinked, but this was how I felt at the time and was afraid to tell him about the elephant in the room.

Frank spent about two hours fitting me on my Fuji track bike – A friend of mine had kindly brought this bike back from New Zealand after picking it up from my brother in law, Alistair, while she was at the rugby world cup over there. It was slightly too big for me and the plan was to get another bike at some stage but I really liked it and it was perfect for the time being. Frank spent about two hours doing the whole fitting. He changed saddle height, altered the angle of my handlebars, added small lifts to my shoes changed the angle of my pedals and so on. He made so many small adjustments I wouldn't even remember them afterwards. He then videoed me on the bike before and after so I could see the difference. I didn't need to see it I could feel it straight away. I instantly felt more powerful on the bike and that it fit me better. It felt great. I felt I had more power in my legs. I was absolutely dying to get it out on the track and try it again – it felt like a new bike! I knew the chances of this happening weren't too likely for a while as no one was going to let me ride the track when it opened again in March and I would be heavily pregnant, but it really gave me something to look forward to. It also gave me the feeling that the Masters, though still very far away, was a reality.

Frank said that when I got a new track bike I could bring it out to him and that we could easily tweak a few adjustments and he'd have it perfect for me in no time. At this point Hugh mentioned to him he had his eye on a bike for me which he thought would be coming available soon. He was trying to persuade Sinéad Jennings, one of the girls on the Irish Team Pursuit squad, to sell me her track bike. Hugh knew that after the girls had been unlucky and missed their chance to qualify for the Olympics, Sinéad was planning on turning all her attentions back to rowing full time and leaving the track cycling behind her so he asked her to give us first refusal. Frank asked him the details of the bike and he reckoned it would be the perfect size for me. I was pretty excited at the thoughts of this – with a bit of luck I'd have a bike that had been ridden by an elite athlete and one of the best female track cyclists in Ireland. Surely that would make me go faster!

The bike became a reality shortly after. Around two months later, I got word from Hugh that Sinead was selling her track bike and some other gear. I was delighted. Hugh delivered it to me one day during his lunch break. I knew I wouldn't be able to ride it until after the birth, but it was super to have it in the house to motivate me. I frequently went out to the shed to inspect it and spent ages admiring it. I instantly loved it. It had arrived in several pieces and required assembly. I decided to do it myself, which took an age and required several phone calls to my brother Dave in Australia who's a pretty handy bike mechanic, explains things with lots of patience and was free to consult on Skype. It was a bit of hassle getting it right, even though track bikes are pretty simple, but with Dave's help I managed. It was worth it in the end to see the finished article. When I stood back and admired my handiwork I had a feeling that this bike was special and would do great things for me. Sounds crazy, but there was something magic about it. Or maybe I just liked the colour – it had a grey carbon finish with blue and shocking pink stripes. I put it at the back of the shed to await its unveiling later in the summer.

During the second trimester I felt more able for exercise then during the first. My energy levels were back a bit closer to normal and most days I felt pretty good and had plenty of energy for training. I did, however, still struggle occasionally with the motivational side of things, especially when going to the gym, as I would often only get the chance to do that late in the evening after a long day at work. I was working three to four days a week at this point and the workload was substantial. Since there were only we two fish vets in the country, it could get pretty busy. There was plenty of trucking all over the country to the different farm sites, mostly in remote locations on the west coast.

In summary, my physical activity during the second trimester consisted of about 8-10 hours training a week. This time consisted mostly of gym sessions and one or two long cycles. Sometimes I managed to turn the travel and nights away that were part of my job to my advantage, staying in a hotel with a gym so I could get a workout in. My exercise volume was at its highest during this time, but the overall intensity was lower than the first trimester. I was also running for variety once or twice a week but was finding this increasingly irritating for one reason in particular, I felt I needed to pee every 5 minutes. I was in and out of the bushes like a yo-yo, and embarrassingly got caught in mid-stream on one occasion. Thankfully the poor witness turned a blind eye however the same couldn't be said for his dog, who found this unusual territory marking by a two legged creature fascinating!

SUSIE MITCHELL

THIRD TRIMESTER – SECOND WIND

I found the transition from the second to the third trimester wasn't as dramatic or noticeable as it had been from the first to the second. What I was doing training-wise didn't change much as a result either. I suppose the start of the second trimester is generally marked for most women by an end to that unsettling, nauseous feeling, which coincides with the time the body has completed its adaptions to the suite of physiological changes that accompany pregnancy. It's more of a slow progression from the second to the third – slowly getting bigger, and finding it gradually harder to squeeze into the same clothes and getting around without feeling like an elephant.

I had planned to stop cycling on the road near the start of the third trimester, around week 30, but this milestone came and went. Even though I had originally planned to give up the open road at this point I didn't want to stop. Hugh's friend had said that by 30 weeks most people have grown quite big and their bumps protrude a lot, so there is less protection for the baby should one be unlucky enough to fall. However, when I hit thirty weeks, my bump was still really small and not really protruding at all. This coupled with the fact that I was enjoying my long spins with coffee stops way to much meant I kept cycling. I didn't really mean to, but things were going so well and I was feeling good so I drifted along into and through the third trimester. I discussed whether I should continue with Hugh, and he made the point that I would never really know what spin would have to be my last and I should just play it by ear and keep it going as long as I felt good and was enjoying myself. I thought this was a good idea.

I suppose as pregnancy progresses through the later stages, anything can happen. I knew, that at any time, some type of pregnancy complication could put an end to my activity, so every extra spin was a bonus. The weather was exceptionally good too for the time of year, and I was making the most of the spins in the fresh air. I also found the bike completely negated the extra weight from the pregnancy making cycling a liberating form of transport. Sometime afterwards, when I asked Hugh what he thought about my performance or physical condition during this time he replied:

"I used to forget you were pregnant. Even though I was aware of all our safe guards, when we were on a spin we never talked about it. We spent most of the time talking about racing and tactics and other bike-related stuff. I would sometimes get a surprise when we would stop for a coffee and I'd notice you were pregnant. Near the end you were starting to go better too and I actually think you were starting to reap the benefits of all the training you had done up to this point, and the fitness you had worked on in the early stages of your pregnancy was coming though. You were getting stronger on the bike. Even though we never pushed it and always rode at your pace, I noticed our easy average speed was back up around 26-27 km/hour."

As I reflected on that time myself, I realised he was right. I felt like I was getting a new lease of life again in the third trimester. I suppose since the body has probably completely adapted to the cardiovascular changes it was reaping the benefits of some of these changes. I discovered Dr Clapp has of course some research to back this up. Regular exercise during pregnancy induces an increase in alveolar ventilation (the amount of air in the lungs available for gas exchange) and the oxygen transfer at a tissue level improves above normal. In addition, peak ventilation (breathing) and maximal aerobic capacity are maintained. By the third trimester the body has adapted to the increased circulatory demands. The feeling of breathlessness common in earlier pregnancy is reduced so these positive effects are really felt. Particularly when the extra weight is negated as it is on the bike. In his book, Dr Clapp described a study he was performing on women who maintained a high level of athletic performance during pregnancy, right through the last trimester. In many instances these women felt so good physically Dr Clapp and his team had to hold them back to prevent them exceeding the amount of exercise required by the protocol or they would have messed up the study. I could totally relate to these women - I just felt stronger as I got towards the end. This is a time a lot of women seem to complain about having no energy and slowing down. I did feel like this sometimes due to the increase in my weight and size, but when I was exercising I felt great. The bike and gym machines like the cross trainer were super for this stage because your weight really doesn't matter that much.

Combining all the cardiovascular changes that occur during pregnancy with training has an interesting side effect down the line post birth. Dr

Clapp found the combination of training and pregnancy increases maximal aerobic capacity (VO_2 max) by 5 – 10 %. This particular effect or *training effect* of pregnancy is usually most apparent six months to one year after the birth. This may be the reason why there are frequently reports of women with significantly improved performance in sport after having a baby. "Brilliant!" I mused. "I might have something to look forward to once I get my body back!"

As I said earlier, one of the reasons I kept riding on the road was because I didn't get very big. In fact I was told repeatedly by people that I had the smallest bump they had ever seen! To the point where I was almost developing a complex about it. At this stage I was going to the antenatal clinic for scans every three weeks or so as is common near the end of pregnancy. I would dread that conversation as I sat in line to see the obstetrician with all the other moms in waiting.

"Is this your first?" it would start. "Yes." "How far along are you?" "Thirty-four weeks." "Oh my God!!! You're joking! That's the smallest bump I've ever seen!" Depending on who I was talking to or how much they probed, I'd furtively say "My mum was like this to, its genetic" (which was actually partly true) or "I'm pretty fit, do a lot of core work and my abs never split apart". Then to defuse the disgust at that I'd follow it with "I've terrible heartburn you know – a bump like this puts awful pressure on your stomach." When they heard this they usually sympathised, glad to hear that I was suffering from something and wasn't just having an easy ride with such a small bump.

The real reason that I remained so small all the way to the end was the fact I didn't develop what's called a *diastasis recti*. I understand that this is something that happens to most women. Basically, during pregnancy the connective tissue in the middle of your abdominal muscles splits apart and relaxes, to make room for the growing baby. The more this happens the more your bump protrudes out the front. I think one of the reasons I didn't get a diastasis was because I worked my core all the way through my pregnancy and my abdominal muscles retained their strength. Maybe if I had got a diastasis I wouldn't have had all that heartburn. If the topic wasn't the size of my bump, the women in the clinic would generally go back to complaining about all sorts of ailments - a common one was how they couldn't turn over in the bed and couldn't sleep on their sides because they were too big - I really felt lucky listening to some of the stories.

I couldn't get over it but so many of the expectant mothers were either overweight or even bordering on obese. It wasn't just large bumps, it was what was around, below, over and under the bumps that was the problem. I encountered a few girls who had been diagnosed with gestational diabetes, a form of diabetes that can occur during pregnancy. I read afterwards that the incidence of this disease has increased in Ireland by 50% in the last 10 years. The increase is largely due to the high number of moms-to-be that are overweight. However, even if these women are overweight when they get pregnant, there is something that can be done to minimise the risk of this form of diabetes. Regular exercise during pregnancy actually increases insulin sensitivity, thereby preventing glucose tolerance problems and gestational diabetes. How many of the women know this I wondered. One girl I was chatting to who had developed this form of diabetes hadn't even been told to exercise by her doctor, even though she was significantly overweight. "I wasn't used to exercise so the doctor told me not to start", she reckoned. I couldn't believe it.

There is no evidence to say that women who never exercised before shouldn't start during pregnancy. This is another misconception that seems quite widespread, even among those who consider themselves in the know. People were always saying to me, "It's OK for you, you're used to it", when they found out how much exercise I was doing at different stages. In his book, Dr Clapp reports his findings from a preliminary study on women who started exercise for the first time during pregnancy. He found that there were no detrimental effects, to the contrary most of the women improved their fitness and definitely their sense of general well-being. By chatting to the other pregnant women over the weeks I attended the clinic, I discovered very few were doing any significant exercise. Some were doing a bit of swimming or yoga or walking. Apart from the odd girl who was sport mad and similar to myself, it seemed hardly any of them were meeting even the basic conservative requirements suggested by ACOG – the 30 minutes of moderate intensity exercise five times per week. It was a real eye-opener.

Around this time I decided to carry out a short survey to gauge the attitudes of recent mothers to exercise during pregnancy. I used the survey tool, SurveyMonkey to do this. I also wanted to know who if anyone had advised them about exercise during this time and what they had been told to do. There were some interesting results. In total nearly 300 women took my survey. I discovered that even though most were in favour of exercising during pregnancy, they nearly all thought that the duration and intensity should be reduced. Another interesting thing I uncovered is that the majority of respondents had been given either no advice re exercise, or in the cases where people had received advice, it was, apart from a few exceptions, quite conservative. It became very clear to me from the survey that every pregnancy was different too. Some women had exercised substantially during their first pregnancy and suffered from terrible complications during the second or third pregnancy to the point where they could hardly walk to the shop. I also came across stories of women desperate to keep going with their exercise regime but with awful side effects that prevented them doing anything. It was interesting to see such a range of experiences.

Around the middle of my third trimester, when I was seven months pregnant, Hugh had another one of his surprises for me to keep me motivated. He arrived at the gym one evening with a lovely skin suit for me in the Sundrive colours. I had always wanted a skin suit but had put it out of my head due to the pregnancy. A skin suit is a tight fitting all in one cycling suit that minimises aerodynamic drag. It's an important piece of kit for the track where seconds are crucial, particularly for anyone who wants to ride in an indoor velodrome. I spent the evening admiring it and imagining that it wouldn't be long until I was wearing it and hopefully fitting into it! It was another one of those things that just gave me that extra boost I needed to keep motivated and keep myself on track for training for the Masters in October.

There were other ways I kept my focus on this goal too. One method was to tell anyone who broached the topic of cycling with me at all about my plans to ride in the Masters in October 2012. Of course I wasn't sure I could make it happen or that there would be any point in going. Even though I was doing all this training, I had absolutely no idea what shape I'd be in four months after giving birth. However, it helped me during that time to say it to different people, reaffirming my plan in my head. Some looked in disbelief with raised eyebrows thinking I was mad. Others never doubted me and were very supportive. I remember in particular a Skype call to my Spanish friend Gonzalo during the later stages of my pregnancy. When I told him my plan he didn't hesitate for a second. "You can do it Susie – no problem for you of all people, you will go kick some ass!" He was so sure, I actually believed him.

Nearing the end of my third trimester I was legally required to stop working, two weeks before I was due. I was a little glad in a way as my boss had long since stopped sending me out to the seawater sites unless the net pens were close enough that I could swim to shore in the event of going into an early labour and I was getting bored of being treated with kid gloves. As the baby ended up being nearly two weeks late this meant I had a month off before the birth, pottering around the house. I know I should have probably been "nesting" but I had to keep up my training or I would have gone mad sitting at home. The weather was actually pretty good in May and that gave me all sorts of options. I was still going on my road bike spins thinking this might be my last one. But it never happened.

One sunny morning in May I went for a spin with Hugh. We met outside the city so we could start cycling directly on quieter country roads, reducing the risk of having to negotiate any traffic. I remember that day well, it was a perfect day for cycling. It was a Saturday morning, the sun was shining and loads of people were out spinning around the roads of North County Dublin. We stopped in our usual coffee spot after about 30km and as I munched on my scone I mentioned to Hugh that it was actually my due date. I wasn't really worried I'd go into labour or anything due to my mother's tardiness with my brothers and I, she was two weeks late delivering all of us. "What?" he said, getting a bit of a shock, "Ok finish that scone, were going back and really, I think we better stop at this point, this is your last spin. You're just pushing it now". He was right I suppose, and in good conscience I couldn't really expect anyone to take the responsibility anymore of going cycling with an overdue pregnant woman! I cycled 50km that day and felt great.

That was the end to all my spinning round the countryside so I had to find an alternative to prevent myself going insane with boredom at home. At this stage I was off work for two weeks and was getting sick of waiting around. My exercise sessions had kept me going. I transferred my efforts to spinning classes in the gym down the road and swimming and weights. I was kind of enjoying going to the gym and lifting weights while so visibly pregnant – I always got a few astonished looks. No-one ever said anything to me like "You shouldn't be doing that", which was nice, people were very encouraging. I particularly enjoyed doing the squats and was able for them as I had maintained the core strength required right through my pregnancy. The planks had only got slightly harder as I got bigger but there wasn't that much of a difference.

Spinning became my way of replacing the road spins during this period. I had been going spinning occasionally throughout the pregnancy when the weather was too bad and it was unsafe for me to ride outside. It became a regular fixture though close to the end when I was overdue. A spin class was fun, had lots of people, good music and it's practically impossible to sit on a bike in that environment and not be motivated. I would inform the instructor before the class commenced that I was pregnant, which was pretty obvious, but would tell them I was doing my own thing. The instructors were really encouraging and supportive once they knew I had been training throughout the pregnancy and trusted me to not do anything stupid. It was funny when they would ask me when I was due as the answer was invariably in the past, like "yesterday" or "last Thursday" I'd follow what the class was doing but keep it in my comfort zone, but still did plenty to get a sweat up. It never ceases to amaze me when you look around a spinning class and there's always a few girls caked in make-up who never sweat!

One particular day when I was about a week overdue the weather was fantastic and I couldn't bear to be inside. I really wanted to ride my bike and I drove out to Corcaigh park. This is a public park on the outskirts of Dublin with a purpose built high quality cycle track about a mile in length. Very safe, nice and smooth and close to the city should anything happen. I did about 20 laps that day and was sorry I hadn't thought of it sooner - it was a great way to get some outdoor exercise at the end.

One of the worst things to happen to me in the last trimester was I picked up a terrible cold. I had been doing so well. Not so much as a sniffle for the whole pregnancy to that point. I was attributing my good health to all the exercise I was doing. In his book, Dr Clapp reported that the incidence of colds and chest infections was much lower in pregnant women who exercise then those who don't. The only problem is when you are unlucky enough to contract something you can't get rid of it, as the immune system is slightly depressed during pregnancy. To make matters worse, you can't take any decent drugs for it either. Around 29 weeks I contracted a nasty head cold, which of course I ignored and continued training. Then the head cold became a chest infection. I believe now had I backed off for a few days I would have saved myself a lot of hardship. I battled through for a week but wasn't getting any better and started coughing up all sorts of green phlegm and ended up on a course of antibiotics. Thankfully the antibiotics cleared up the secondary infection and I improved, but I had to stay completely off the bike and out of the gym for about 10 days in the end. The remnants of the cold lingered for a few weeks afterwards which for me was very unusual. I'm rarely sick and never for long. It was part and parcel of pregnancy I suppose. The whole way through the pregnancy I had been trying to optimise my immunity and was eating pretty well along with religiously taking "Pregnacare" vitamin supplements and extra vitamin C. I found these supplements really good, as they were balanced and didn't overdose you on anything, which can be dangerous for the baby. In terms of sport-specific nutrition I had never been a massive fan of purpose designed energy drinks and supplements, but however I did have a fondness for a particular recovery drink, which I would usually consume after a long spin or a gym session. I continued with this supplement even though very little research had been performed on these supplements and how they might affect pregnancy, I checked the ingredients and felt that it was safe enough. The supplement, called '2:1:1 Recovery' is made by Optimum Nutrition, and its main protein components are whey, casein and egg albumen and the carbohydrate components mostly glucose and fructose. I'd also seen pregnant women put a lot worse into their bodies with no apparent ill effects.

So I continued with my exercise, biking, spinning classes at my own speed, swimming and strength and conditioning right through the end of the third trimester and past it once my due date came and went. In that period after I was due I spent most days waiting around for something to happen. It was really frustrating at times. I'd go down to the gym and one of the girls who worked there would say "No baby yet then?" or "Are you still here?" when I was about ten days over. I even turned to the internet in search of natural remedies to help kick start labour. Disappointed, I discovered most of the things that are supposed to bring on labour are actually only old wives tales or urban myths. From spicy food to brisk walking, sex to acupressure, it had all been tested by science and nothing seemed to really work. The only natural remedy that was given any kudos by science was taking a large dose of castor oil, the dose was 60mls mixed with orange juice to give this vile oil a more pleasant flavour. What this tasty concoction does is basically gives you a large dose of diarrhoea and bowel cramping. This violent assault on your digestive system sets off a cascade of physical and neurological effects which can trigger labour. I considered it for a nanosecond but didn't think it would be worth it. It could be dangerous too and there were reports of people ending up seriously dehydrated – the last thing one needs when entering a labour marathon. I asked my obstetrician about the castor oil and he told me they actually used to use castor oil enemas to induce labour before all the modern drugs became available. I decided it was all a bit to unpleasant and I'd bide my time and wait for things to happen naturally.

SUSIE MITCHELL

BIRTH AND POST-PARTUM RETURN TO EXERCISE

Like so many other expectant mothers my vision of the birth of my baby and what actually happened were two completely separate entities. I wanted more than anything to have a natural labour with no intervention whatsoever – no inductions, epidurals or pain relief, no forceps or suction, no stiches post-delivery. No, none of the above was in my birth plan. I was so fit I hoped I could cope with everything Mother Nature threw at me. When I sat through my antenatal class and people were asking about epidurals and other pain relief I sat back. I had no intention of getting an epidural or taking any sort of pain relief. I was sure I wouldn't opt for it no matter what. In hindsight though and from talking to loads of other mums, I really think that's a decision a woman can only make on the day. A lot of people who don't want any pain relief opt for it and vice versa.

Anyway, I was pretty confident that my labour would go smoothly and my biggest worry was how I was going to minimise the possibility of getting a perineal tear and avoid getting stiches as both would delay my return to the bike. I had read it could take up to six weeks or more to sit on the saddle again with a bad tear. I had also read that cyclists were actually more prone to getting tears during delivery as their perineum was a bit "saddle-hardened" and not as flexible as non-cyclists! I had therefore employed my husband as full time perineal masseuse. I won't go into to detail on what was involved, except to say it wasn't anywhere near as enjoyable as a back, neck and shoulder massage. However, I felt it was worth the effort, as perineal massage was supposed to significantly reduce the chances of stiches, in particular if it was your first baby. There! I had ticked all the boxes. That was everything sorted. I laugh at my naivety as I write this afterwards because this was actually my only big concern at the time. I gave absolutely no thought to the fact that I was about to get the biggest shock of my life – responsibility for another human being.

At my 36 week check I discovered my baby was in transverse lie, which of course wasn't part of the plan. If this position failed to correct itself, I was looking at being scheduled in for a caesarean section – something I really didn't want. I heard that doing some inversions, basically hanging head down off the edge of the couch could help a baby correct its position so I employed this strategy and to my surprise it seemed to work. After a few days of these of trying, there was an almighty heave as we were watching TV one evening. "Did you see that?" I said to Cormac and I watched my stomach develop a life of its own. That scene from the movie Alien came to mind, just before the baby alien popped out of John Hurt's stomach! Cormac was amazed. "I'm pretty sure that was the baby turning around", I said. On the next scan at 38 weeks the baby was indeed head down and ready to go. Thankfully, my perfect birth plan was back on track.

My due date came and went with no sign of any baby arriving. Clearly no one had told the baby about it. I expected to be a bit late as my mother had also been, but I was hoping for no more than a week overdue because I had read that exercising mothers deliver on average a week earlier than non-exercising mothers (I subsequently found this statistic only referred to women participating in high impact sports such as running or aerobics). D-day for an induction was fast approaching. In my hospital you were allowed to go the full two weeks overdue, as long as a 12-day scan indicated there were no complications. When I got to day ten overdue I was really starting to get annoyed with the whole thing. I wanted a natural birth and the baby, it seemed, had no intention of showing face. I spoke with my sister-in-law and she suggested I try acupuncture. I found a clinic to attend in the city centre. I was ready to try anything.

I wasn't sure I believed acupuncture would work but having had it before for an injury I knew it was pretty relaxing and reckoned it would do no harm. When I arrived, one of the first things the acupuncturist asked me what condition my cervix was in. I thought this was a bit of an odd question. "What?!" I said, wondering if I had misheard her. "You know, how many centimetres are you dilated?" she asked me. I didn't have a clue and nearly laughed. "Sure how would I know?" I asked her completely baffled, "No one's had a look. Am I supposed to be able to feel it or something?" She was shocked and went on a complete rant about it. She lectured me so much I started to grow worried. She made me feel like that something was wrong with the fact that no one had been poking and prodding at me down there. The outcome was that without knowing the condition of said cervix she informed me she couldn't stick a needle in the key point that would kick off labour, which in hindsight was possibly a good thing. She was able to find other places to stick the needles though and after turning me into a pin cushion she left the room and I lay there relaxing. Lying there with nothing to do but chill, I kind of noticed that the baby's movements seemed to sort of reduced somewhat. I could still feel her fluttering around inside but there was a subtle difference, the movements were not as strong or abrupt as before. It was hard to call though as I was getting a lot of Braxton Hicks contractions. These are false contractions that are not painful they just feel like a wave of tightening across your abdomen. I worried though as there did seem to be a subtle difference. Suddenly as if in response to my worry I got a good kick from inside and felt reassured. That night as I lay in bed I worried again about the baby's movements. Again, it was subtle but there was definitely a difference to the way they had been a few days previous. We had been informed in our antenatal class that to get ourselves to the hospital for a check-up if the baby's movements stopped at any stage. The midwife giving the class told an awful story at the time of a lady who was very close to her due date when the baby had gone quiet. She rang her sister and a friend, both of whom told her it was normal for the movements to diminish towards the end. The baby was stillborn shortly after. This horror story had stuck with me and I hummed and hawed about going to the hospital. Cormac reassured me that everything would be fine and we were going to the hospital in the morning for my 12-day overdue scan and could get it fully checked out then. I relaxed a bit and went asleep.

The following morning I felt a little gush of water as I jumped out of bed which turned out to be quite blood stained. I wondered was this the start of it all and was a bit worried about the blood. After a large breakfast, anticipating a potentially long day ahead, we headed to the hospital for my scan. The room was full of moms-to-be when I arrived, waiting around for their scans. As I checked in at the desk I mentioned I was concerned that things were not quite right. I was whisked aside immediately and fast tracked and within a few minutes I was having an ultrasound. On examination, there was still plenty of fluid around the baby, and it did appear to be moving. "Looks fine", the girl performing the scanning smiled and as the baby waved an arm said, "We'll get the doctor to see you now". I was relieved. However, it still just didn't feel quite right. A lovely young registrar called Mark came in to check me out. Inspired by the crazy acupuncture lady the previous day and also curious, I asked him could he check the condition of my cervix to see if I had any chance of going into labour anytime soon. He obliged. "No sign of it being anywhere near favourable. I'm afraid were going to have to book you in for an induction first thing in the morning. I will give you tonight to labour yourself but I'm pretty sure we'll see you back tomorrow at 8am". "I won't lie to you", he continued. "Induction isn't pleasant. I have had plenty women say to me they would come back for another natural birth or even come back for another caesarean, but no one would come back voluntarily for an induction". Much as I didn't want it I accepted that induction was going to be my fate but still couldn't shake the feeling there was something amiss. As I was about to leave I told Mark even though the ultrasound scan indicated the baby was fine, I felt the movements had significantly reduced. When he heard this he gave me a studied look and paused for a second. I could see his brain ticking over. "I'm sure there will be nothing to worry about but we'll just do a quick trace on the foetal heart rate to check that everything is OK before you go". It turned out he had pretty good instincts.

A female paediatrician took over from Mark a few minutes later and as she hooked me up to the monitor she explained "we are recording two things here, the heart rate of the foetus and also your uterine tone. As you can see here were getting a really nice trace on those Braxton Hicks contractions you're having – God you've great abdominal tone! On a lot of women we can't even pick up these uterine movements." Another advantage of the core work I had been doing! As I sat there a pattern began to emerge. Every Braxton Hicks was followed by a big reduction in the foetal heart rate with it dropping from a normal 140 beats per minute down to 70-80. Then it would recover again. The paediatrician came back after 15 minutes to check the trace – "See what's happening here?", as she pointed to the trace, "These dips in heart rate are known as late decelerations – and they are a significant cause for concern. They indicate the foetus in in distress. I think there may be a problem with the cord". Mark was there to. "We will have to bring you upstairs immediately and break your waters", he said." I couldn't believe it. I was terrified, my heart was pounding – this was it! And I wasn't ready. And what if there was something wrong with my baby? Within five minutes I was lying on a bed upstairs surrounded by people. Another consultant obstetrician took over. Mark explained that it was going to be tricky to break my waters with my unfavourable cervix and he was letting someone else who was more experienced run the gauntlet on this one. "Great", I thought, "this is clearly going to be fun." My new obstetrician sat down on the bed and looked at the heart rate trace from the machine for about two seconds before he said to the nurses, "Prep her for a section". Then he turned to me and said abruptly "In case we have to do a general anaesthetic, have you had anything to eat today?" He was less than impressed when I told him about the large breakfast I had consumed only two hours before.

The nurses went about their business and before I knew it my clothes were pulled off and bundled into a plastic sack and handed to Cormac, my bikini line was shaved and a blood sample had been taken from my right arm. Then the obstetrician went about breaking my waters, which wasn't too pleasant as it took a number of digs with the plastic hook before he could manage to rupture the membranes. Not an experience I'd care to repeat any time soon. Eventually after what felt like an age although probably only two or three minutes, I felt a massive warm gush and he said, "MEC 2 to 3 – get her to theatre now". This meant there was meconium present in the amniotic fluid at levels bad enough to warrant an emergency section. Meconium is a foetal waste product and its presence indicated the foetus was in significant distress. I was shaking like a leaf at this point. Everything was becoming a blur. Within a matter of minutes I was numb from the chest down with the spinal anaesthetic. It was such an odd sensation, and a bit frightening. The surgery began with lightning speed and I could feel pressure and people pulling at my abdomen, but no pain. A lovely easy-going calm surgeon had taken over from the evil water-breaking man. Within about four minutes of starting he had incised into the womb and was inspecting the baby in situ. "There's the problem. The cord is wrapped around the neck tightly three times". Watching his reflection in the overhead theatre lights, I could see him unwinding something. Next thing I knew I felt an almighty sense of relief in my abdomen – like someone had released a pressure valve or something – it was such a bizarre sensation and a massive relief and came about as they lifted the baby out. It felt like my stomach was having an out of body experience.

Everything happened so quickly. I could see them lifting out a spindly looking baby with long arms and legs. They suctioned her lungs before stimulating her to breathe in case there was any meconium aspiration, which thankfully there wasn't. She was examined by a paediatrician and within five minutes given a full bill of health and brought over to me wrapped in a blue blanket so I could see her. I was overcome with relief. We had a beautiful healthy 6lb baby girl! I couldn't touch her as my arms were stuck under the surgical drapes so had a sniff of her skin as the nurse put her up against my face. She was like a tiny doll. Cormac was allowed to hold her. After being stitched up and before I went to recovery they allowed me to breast feed her for ten minutes. I marvelled at how strong the suck reflex was on such a tiny thing and how she knew exactly what to do while I was completely clueless. Then Cormac took her away to mind her while I was in recovery. He had enjoyed the whole thing and had taken pictures with his iPhone. At one stage when I was under the knife he asked if he could have a look and stood up to peer over the drape curtain – he nearly passed out. I think it was the metal retractors pulling my abdominal muscles apart that made him feel a bit ill!

So, as I said the best laid plans for the birth went to waste. I was actually very fortunate that I hadn't laboured myself because there could then have been a very serious situation. The false contractions had produced a substantial worrying reduction in foetal heart rate and I couldn't help but wonder what impact real labour contractions would have had. The surgeon called in to the ward to see me after I had been brought down from recovery. He basically informed me there was no way the baby would have survived a natural delivery with so much cord wrapped around her neck – not to mention the foetal distress that would have occurred as a result of proper labour contractions. I felt fortunate indeed to have been in Holles Street, which is the National Maternity Hospital, surrounded by such a team of experienced and competent doctors and midwives. Much as I had liked the idea of no intervention, I was so grateful for it. If it had been 50 years ago there's no doubt my story would not have had such a happy ending.

I had to spend five days in hospital after the surgery. It was great to have the support and advice of the nurses and doctors there in my first few days of motherhood. I had time to marvel at how beautiful my baby girl was, and couldn't help but feel she was a little miracle. We decided to call her Tori, a name picked by my husband years before, should he ever have a girl. I liked it too, as it was simple but still a little unusual.

Having a section wasn't something I had ever considered so I had never thought about how it would affect my exercise and training plans. Despite the joy of having Tori around, I had no choice but to face up to it as I lay in the hospital bed the day after the surgery in a lot of pain and discomfort. The day after a section is particularly painful as what often happens is a lot of air gets trapped in your abdomen during surgery and you have these shooting pains up and down your body as a result. My shoulders were more painful than where the incision site was. "There goes my plans to get out of hospital and straight back on the bike", I thought. I had planned, that all going well with my lovely natural birth and no perineal tears and so on, that I would be back training within ten days. This seemed to be the minimum number of days before athletes I had read about or talked to returned to training. I thought if things were really bad, the most awful thing I would have to worry about was a few stiches in my perineum. I worried how this might affect my sitting on the bike saddle and if it would greatly delay my return. However, what had happened meant that I wasn't recovering from a normal delivery. I was now recovering from major abdominal surgery, not to mention the other after effects of having a baby. Severe hormonal changes, sleep deprivation and the most difficult part - trying to get your head around responsibility for a new human being for the foreseeable future. I can honestly say getting to grips with all this meant the next ten days to two weeks were probably the hardest of my life.

I had made so many plans about what the birth would be like and how I would return to exercise afterwards, I had never thought about the fact that I was going to experience a major life change. I didn't realise the psychological impact that becoming a parent was going to have on me. I thought that my biggest worry would be finding time to get out and exercise, in reality my biggest problem was dealing with what was going on in my mind. I finally realised that when people said you don't know what's ahead of you, this was what they meant. I couldn't believe how it felt to be a parent, to all of a sudden be responsible for someone else with no way out and every decision I made and thing I wanted to do would be in part dictated by them from now on. I found the responsibility quite overwhelming. I went from feeling really down in the dumps and trapped, to feeling guilty for having these thoughts. I found myself actually in mourning for my life before the baby. I would see people cycling past my window going about their daily lives and I was jealous – the freedom to be able to do such things. I knew I should be happy as I had a healthy baby girl. I could have had one with all sorts of problems or none at all had the birth not gone so well in the end. I had heard from everyone about this overwhelming love you feel for your baby, like nothing you ever experienced. Where were these feelings? I felt wretched for not having them instantly as I thought I should and not taking to motherhood like it was the best thing that ever happened to me, as I perceived so many women had done before me. After I came out of these doldrums I realised I did of course love Tori, but it was such a huge adjustment for me and the way of thinking I normally employed that the whole experience completely floored me. The hormone withdrawal was of course probably also playing its part in the way I was feeling. I had heard that sometimes the hormonal effects post-partum can be worse if you have a C-section as opposed to going through a normal labour. Perhaps this contributed to the blues I was feeling. I had also heard about post-partum depression and how it affects up to one in ten women – the thoughts that my baby blues would develop into this terrified me too. When I read back on this now, months later, I'm so glad I wrote about how I was feeling at the time. I wrote this chapter about three weeks post-partum when the experience was fresh in my mind. If I were trying to recall this period now I would definitely do so with rose tinted glasses. I remember being particularly down in the dumps one day, when I found a chapter that really helped in one of the books I had purchased about pregnancy and exercise. It was quite an old book, about running during pregnancy and post-partum and had been written in a personal style much like this book. The author talked about how hard those first few weeks were, what she went through and how normal that was. I devoured that chapter and re-read it. It really helped me to find someone out there had experienced the same thing. That's why I wanted to really write honestly about how it was for me, so maybe I could help someone else when they read my words.

Around this time I also talked to a few good friends of mine who had babies, which also helped make things a little easier. Niamh, a girl I had known since early schooldays right through sharing a flat in college was particularly sympathetic. She had two kids so was ahead of me in the game but was really able to empathise with me having been through it all herself. I would urge anyone if they are finding things hard at the start to talk to someone – sometimes that's all you need to feel better, a chance to be honest about how you're feeling and for someone to understand.

After what were probably the longest two weeks of my life, I found I started to feel slightly better. As the fog cleared, I slowly started to cope. I could look a little into the future again without freaking out. The best piece of advice I got during this period was from a friend John, who had recently had a baby himself. He advised us to take any help that is offered from anyone. I remember my mother-in-law, Anne, came up to stay with us two weeks after the birth and offered to mind the baby for a night just to give us a good night's sleep. I couldn't believe she was prepared to do it but took her up on the offer. I think this was the turning point for me. It's amazing how the world can appear to be a better place when you have a night of uninterrupted sleep. I think it was probably the best baby present anyone gave me. All of a sudden things were bearable. Yes it was still hard from day to day but I was coping much better mentally.

Another plan that hadn't rolled out as well as I had wanted was the one where I was going to feed the baby myself for six months. Breast feeding had posed a major challenge for me. I was a mess. I seemed to be breast feeding for at least 12 out of every 24 hours. What had started so well in the hospital went seriously downhill after a week. I had seemed initially to have a great milk supply but it had dwindled significantly by the ten day mark leaving me with a frustrated hungry baby. I'm not sure exactly what went wrong for me but it was probably a combination of a few things. Firstly, calorie restriction may have been responsible. It was not something I had done deliberately. However, while I had eaten rings around myself in the hospital I had lost my appetite since I got home, probably due to exhaustion. In addition to this I had not put on very much weight myself at all during pregnancy. This was probably partly due to all the exercise I was doing, but I had also suffered terribly from heartburn from mid-pregnancy onwards, and this had significantly curtailed my appetite. The second thing I thought may have been responsible was that since returning home I had been going out for pretty long (although meandering) walks every day to get some fresh air which I thought may have had a negative impact on my milk supply. I had anecdotally heard that any activity could affect lactation. When I investigated this further I found that there have been relatively few studies that have actually looked at how maternal exercise or activity levels affect breast feeding. There was a series of studies carried out by a group of nutritionists in California in the 1990s that suggested frequent sustained high-intensity running during lactation did not impair the quantity or the quality of human breast milk. There may have been other factors at play in my case. My gut feeling was that because my body was simultaneously trying to recover from major abdominal surgery, it was possible that it was prioritising its resources into my own recovery instead of lactation. I had thought that having a section would leave me incapacitated and I would be struggling physically for weeks. However, my recovery seemed to be remarkably fast, after that first day of agony. Within a few days, I was off all pain killers and wasn't even getting a twinge. My skin wound was almost fully healed within ten days and I felt strong and had been doing some easy walking after a week or so. Healing post-surgery uses quite a lot of your body's resources so it seems reasonable to deduce that it can have some impact on the supply of breast milk. Finally, in terms of the actual mechanics of breastfeeding, I felt that I possibly had a very slow milk let down reflex and my baby was absolutely exhausting herself trying to fill herself up. I rang the public health nurse on day ten post-partum in tears and she advised me to introduce supplementary bottle feeding if I was worried about the baby not getting enough. So for the next few weeks I did both. This led to a much happier, satisfied baby who was gaining weight, not to mention a much saner satisfied mother who was getting at least a few hours sleep at night now. There was also a bit more freedom not being a permanent milking parlour.

There is huge pressure on mothers today to breastfeed. Yes, it is the best food for your baby, convenient and free. But don't beat yourself up if it doesn't work for you. Formula today is practically identical in nutritional value to breast milk so it's not the end of the world if you have to choose this method of feeding for whatever reason. Transferring the colostrum to your baby over those first few days is one of the most important benefits breastfed babies get so even if you can do that and switch to formula it's great.

I wanted to write about these few weeks post-partum, as I wanted anyone having their first baby to know that things mightn't quite be as you expect, and you need to know it's normal. I also wanted to show that there is light at the end of the tunnel. In the broad sense of things its actually quite a short time until you start to feel normal again, a matter of a few weeks, but when you are in those few weeks it may as well be forever, and it certainly feels like it. I found that most other mothers I spoke to had gone through something similar with their first. The underlying consensus was the first few weeks post-partum after their first baby were some of the hardest of their lives. Of course I'm sure that there are some people out there who take to it like a duck to water but I believe they are the exceptions. I suppose my whole experience was compounded by the fact that I was so active and busy prior to the birth. Hardly a day went by in my life that I didn't undertake some sort of activity, and I had to sustain the longest period in living memory without any exercise, which undoubtedly contributed to my feeling the blues.

My next challenge was to figure out when I could get back on the bike after the surgery. I was starting to see that having a section may have a few advantages. A major one was going to be that sitting on my saddle was no longer an issue. When I investigated the recommendations, everything I read rolled out a standard ban of at least six weeks before you could do anything after a section. This magic number seemed to apply whether it was in relation to driving, exercise, having sex or looking out the window. When return to exercise was mentioned specifically, I saw advice ranging from four to twelve weeks. This was clearly a grey area and I reckoned probably strongly related to the individual in question. From my experience as a veterinary surgeon, I knew something of wound healing and how wound strength progressed over time so decided to make my own informed decision. I knew about 70% of the tensile strength would have returned to most of the abdominal tissues within about three weeks, had the healing gone well and without complications. I also knew the guy who had operated on me was a highly-skilled and experienced surgeon, which makes a big difference. When I quizzed him about his job afterwards I discovered he was doing approximately ten sections a day, and I knew he had worked as an obstetrician for many years up to that point. From my own surgical experience I knew that the better the surgeon the quicker the healing. When I started out as a newly qualified vet and was doing caesarean sections and neutering different animals they sometimes took a little longer to recover and were more prone to post-operative complications than when I became a more experienced surgeon. This is down to two things. Firstly the time it takes to do the surgery is important and you obviously become much quicker with practice, but secondly, it is also due to gentle tissue handling, which is a tacit skill that you only develop through practical experience. A friend of mine also had an emergency section for her first baby and in contrast to me, it had taken her quite a long time to recover. This girl was pretty hardy so I know she wasn't joking when she said she didn't feel right internally when she went running for months after – I suspected she may have suffered a lot of adhesions as a result of the surgery. Perhaps this was due to chance, but it also may have been because she had her baby in a really small hospital where the obstetricians might be relatively inexperienced, only doing a handful of sections a week. Not like the National Maternity Hospital, the veritable baby factory where I had Tori.

Armed with this knowledge about my own healing, in combination with my pending insanity if I didn't get out and do something, I tentatively got back up on the bike two and a half weeks post birth. I got the go ahead from my coach to just roll around, so said goodbye to Cormac and Tori and set off one Saturday morning. When I arrived at the track I had a massive flock of butterflies in my stomach. I didn't know if it was anticipation, excitement or nerves. It wasn't just physical, it was the mental ramifications of doing something which defined who I was again, when there had been nothing but baby 24-7 for what seemed like an eternity. As I readied myself for off, my feet were shaking and I was fumbling with the pedals so much I had to get someone else to help me clip in. Then I pushed off the fence and was rolling. It was a fine summer's day and there was a gentle breeze on my face. I don't think I have ever enjoyed or appreciated riding my bike as much. The sense of freedom was something else and it felt like a momentous occasion to me. After that it was like someone flicked a switch on the back of my head. My mood lifted considerably and I felt like there was some hope of returning to a normal life, obviously a totally different one now that there was another little person involved but that just meant someone new to share my experiences with.

The next day I did an easy 40km spin around the Phoenix Park. The park is one of Dublin's greatest assets. It's the second largest park in a city in Europe and is a lovely, safe place to ride your bike. It's so big you can easily clock up 30-40 km after just a couple of laps. The following evening was a Monday, a track training night, so I was back down there in a flash. On Hugh's advice I participated in the junior session and rode the senior warm up, where I pushed it a little for the first time. It felt good to get the heart rate up a bit again as it had been so long since I had done anything strenuous. I remained very conscious that I was still in recovery from my surgery and didn't go too crazy, but it was just so nice to get a vague idea of where my fitness was at, as you really have no clue what is going to happen post-partum. You don't know what effect any of the training had during your pregnancy or what effect, suddenly not being pregnant again, will have on your fitness. The feeling of being able to cycle comfortably minus bump was a huge relief. That pressure on my stomach was gone and there wasn't a trace of the heartburn that had plagued my pregnancy.

It is really amazing how you slowly adapt to the physical constraints of pregnancy as it progresses and it's only when the bump is gone that you realise how awkward it felt. I found myself again applying the advice I had received at the beginning of pregnancy when trying to gauge my efforts post-partum, "listen to your body". I can't stress how important this piece of advice is. From talking to a lot of people about exercising during their pregnancies, and from my survey, there's one thing I had to acknowledge - everyone is different! Pregnancy affects everyone in different ways, sometimes these differences can be dramatic, as are peoples' experience during birth. People recover at different rates too, so just because I felt well enough to get back on my bike after a few weeks that doesn't mean everyone should be able to. Some women might be back in the saddle even quicker than me. You just have to know your limits and tune into what your body is telling you to do. It will let you know soon enough if you've overstepped the line.

Over the next few weeks, I continued to train slowly building up on volume and intensity. I attended track training sessions whenever I could and participated at a level that I felt comfortable, skipping some drills and doing others. Around the start of week five post-partum, and about two and a half weeks after getting back on the bike, something significant happened – I felt the strength in my legs really returning properly for the first time. I did a session on the rollers in my house and did some easy core work, planks and the likes and felt within touching distance of the ability and strength I once had. There was definitely a subtle shift in how I was feeling and the response of my body to exercise. "I feel strong", I acknowledged to myself, mildly surprised as I was spinning away in time to the music. The following evening I went to the track to do a full senior training session and was rolling pretty well. We even did some sprint efforts near the end of the session and I surprised myself. I wasn't going to break any land speed records that night but my body felt close to normal again. What's more, I could sense the untapped potential that was in there.

RACES & MEDALS WITH BABY ON BOARD

After that senior training session in which I felt so good I cornered Hugh in the clubhouse. I wanted to run something by him. "What do you think of me doing the National Olympic Omnium next weekend?", I asked. He paused for a moment thinking. "You have actually progressed very quickly", he observed. "Yes. Actually I think from what I've seen tonight that wouldn't be a bad idea. You looked strong. Something has changed." So he had noticed it to. "If nothing else it will give us some times in the fixed events to see where we are at for the season ahead and give us something to work on. It will be good all-round experience for you to. Even though your fitness might be challenged in some of the bunch races I think it will be good for you to compete".

The Olympic Omnium is a track event made up of six events and raced over two days. It consists of three individual timed events, the Flying 250m, the Pursuit and the 500m Time Trial, and three bunch races, the Points, Elimination and Scratch. I really wanted to compete in it and felt I was ready to give it a bash. The wonderful thing was that I wouldn't be under any pressure to perform having only returned six weeks after the birth and no one would expect me to do anything of note. Hugh was a little concerned as he didn't want to put me in a situation where I would be beaten by people whom I would normally beat, but this didn't bother me at all – I knew I couldn't really go in with any expectations given the circumstances. I just wanted to get racing again. I did a couple of sessions on the rollers that week in preparation for the event and raced the Wednesday night track league, where I didn't disgrace myself, so with some trepidation was looking forward to the weekend.

The Saturday morning of the Omnium dawned nice and sunny. I was so excited signing on with my licence at the clubhouse. I had another good reason to be happy today too. I was about to ride Sinead Jennings' bike in competition for the first time, and was expecting great things from it. Cormac brought me down to the track and helped me get my stuff set up for the day ahead. He had Tori in her sling and was carrying her around. She was so tiny, I think people who didn't know me were looking at the size of her and wondering whether I had just given birth and whether I was mad to be carting stuff into the track centre and competing. There was a good entry, with 12 women in total. The first event was the Flying 250 which I made a mess of and did a pretty slow time of 19 seconds, which left me seventh overall. "You're entry speed was way too slow, what were you thinking?" Hugh chided, when I got off the track. I wasn't thinking, that was the problem! I was finding it hard to switch myself on to competition again it had been so long. You need to be very, very focussed in the sprint events to get the best of yourself, the shorter the event the more focus required. Anyway Sinead's bike felt good so that was a positive, and I was enjoying riding it. The next race was my least favourite bunch race, the Points Race. This involves riding 20 laps with sprints for points occurring every five laps. I managed to score some points during the first sprint, but went a bit hard and ended up swinging for the rest of the race and just hanging in. Hugh gently pointed out my mistake to me afterwards, but I was pleased as I had at least scored a few points and maintained my seventh position in the rankings. After a short break the next race was the last of the day and my favourite. Even though I really didn't have a clue as I hadn't ridden too many of them, I loved the Elimination Race. It was probably the most technically challenging of the bunch races. The rules of this race are simple, the last person across the line in every lap is out. Hugh pulled me aside beforehand to give me some advice. "The way to ride this race is halfway between the yellow and the blue line and always make sure there is someone below you. Simple as that". As we pulled off from the fence, it seemed that other riders had the same plan as me and I was jostled out of position pretty quickly. I pulled up the track and made another attempt and took up the position a bit more forcefully and this time I held it. Lap after lap we accelerated approaching the line and each time I managed to avoid elimination. Suddenly there were only two of us left! Róisín, one of the other girls who eventually came second overall, beat me in the last lap, but I had ridden well and was delighted. That was probably my best finish in a bunch race on the track ever – not that I had done very many of them. I think that was a pivotal moment for me in the Omnium, and I felt like things were definitely going better than expected. Hugh really wanted me to finish in the top six and I was well positioned for this after day one. He was pleased with my performance. "It's the bike I told him. It knows how to win". I really did feel there was something special about it, I had from the start.

After the usual baby induced sleep deprived night that had become my staple, I got up the next morning for day two. Again the weather was fantastic. The first event that morning was the Individual Pursuit, a 3km timed event. Hugh had told me to try and ride steady, with a measured pace. My experience in the Nationals the previous year had been the opposite. It was the only other time I had ridden a Pursuit in competition and my laps were all over the place. They had gone something like this: very fast, fast, middling, slow, slower and even slower. I had completely burned myself out at the start, having no idea how to ride a Pursuit properly. This time around I was more careful at the start and kept saying the word "measured" to myself as I cranked out the six laps. It worked. My splits were nearly perfect, with every lap taking the same time. I had ridden well within myself and produced a time of 4.30, good enough for third! What's more I was only eight seconds behind Róisín. I was delighted with this as I considered her to be a good rider and was pleased to be so close in time to her. My time in the Nationals the previous year had been 4.34 so 4:30 was a new PB, and because I had technically ridden it better, it had felt nowhere near as hard. I knew I had more in me but would have to put that off for another day.

The next event was the Scratch Race, this was the one I was most worried about. At this stage in an Omnium it can get quite complicated as riders watch those close to them in the rankings, trying to get the better of each other. It changes the dynamics of a race. Hugh explained to me what was likely to happen and gave me a plan. "Sarah and Róisín will be watching each other as both could potentially win gold. The only person you need to worry about is Amy, a pretty strong young rider but she doesn't have much track experience. You need to beat her at all costs. If with three laps to go, no one has made a run for it, you do it. Just don't take her with you". The race went exactly as Hugh described. It was pretty cagey and a lot of eyeballing was going on. I went into autopilot when I came around and saw "3" on the board. I rode up the track to get some height, forcing Amy, who was riding beside me, up to the fence and in the process she kind of got stuck in behind Róisín's wheel. I didn't need an invitation, once I saw that she was out of reach I put the head down and jumped hard off the banking, pumping my legs for all they were worth. I didn't even look up until I had a lap done. When I did I couldn't believe it but there was no one on my wheel. No one had reacted and come with me. All I had to do was hold on for the remaining two laps and it was mine. "Oh shit, I don't think I can hold this", I thought. I was starting to die in the last lap but the adrenalin somehow kept me going. When I crossed the line I punched the air and roared "YES!" It was the first time I had ever won a bunch race, not to mention my performance had just put me in the bronze medal position for the Omnium.

All that was left now was the 500TT and as long as I beat Amy in that I was home and dry. The 500 was one of my favourite events and even though I didn't do a great time in it that day, it was enough. I had beaten Amy by 0.15 of a second and she ended up in 4th and I had won the bronze. I was so thrilled. I absolutely couldn't believe it. I had won a national medal! It was something I never dreamed I could do and not to mention only six weeks after having a baby. I was in a daze. Hugh came over to me and I threw myself at him. "Thank you so much for getting me here," I blubbered, "You have no idea how much this means to me". He did of course though. In fact he knew more than anyone else. For once he was actually stuck for words and went quiet. Eventually afterwards he told me that he thought I was in with a very good chance of winning the bronze at the end of day one. He didn't want to say it to me to put me under pressure but had rung one of the other coaches, Terry, and explained to him exactly how it would happen. Then he rang another rider from the club, Keith, and told him the same. "And it went exactly according to plan, it was clockwork today. I am so happy for you. A National medal. Some riders go their whole lives and never win one of them!" I drove home afterwards in a daze listening to Tiny Tempah's album and that song he does with Kelly Roland was playing "Invincible, Invincible", she sang, I belted it out along with her. I knew the song wasn't about cycling, but I felt pretty invincible at that moment. I didn't know if the whole thing was an accident or whether I'd win again on the track but I was enjoying every moment of it.

I was high as a kite for about two weeks after the Omnium. I had shown I was up for it and a credible rider. Even though I had made the podium, the medal had been won using brains as much as brawn. I knew I was lacking a bit in stamina and base fitness, I could feel it. So I settled in to do some proper training. This wasn't easy to schedule with a small baby and a husband to consider, and the summer became a bit of a juggling act. I have a very understanding husband in Cormac, but his patience was frequently tried by my antics during the next few months. I am a very focussed person when I have a project in hand. My project post baby was, come hell or high water, to get my fitness back and compete in the World Track Masters in Manchester as a credible rider. I wasn't thinking medals, I was thinking quality experience for future years. Realistically, I was looking at October 2012 as an opportunity to lay down some good times to give me something to aim to beat the following year, where I would hopefully have an opportunity to win a medal. My success in the Omnium made me feel for the first time that I wasn't wasting my time planning for the Masters. Even though I knew it might be a few years before I'd potentially win any medals at World Masters level, I felt I could return this year and be at least as good and hopefully a bit better then in 2011, gaining some valuable experience along the way.

Being a full-time mum minding a baby can be pretty time consuming if you let it, but I was determined to get as much quality training in as I could while on maternity leave and turn it to my advantage. I had a few issues though. I couldn't really get out unless Cormac or my mum were there to take over. So I had to find a way of training during the day while Tori slept. That's where the rollers, my trusty stationary trainer came in. I tried to use the rollers on the days I couldn't get out to the track or for a road spin. I took advantage when Cormac came home in the evenings. The summer track training schedule suited our situation, as most of the sessions ran in the evenings from about 6.30 until 8.30. So as poor Cormac would arrive home from work I would meet him in the doorway and hand over baby Tori, and slip out past him with my track bike and gear bag on my shoulder and head off for the evening. I tried to get out for long spins with the Sundrive crew at the weekends but whatever about the evening sessions, I think Cormac found these stints particularly hard to deal with. I'd arrive home after being gone from 9am until 1pm and he would say "Where were you? I have been stuck with the baby on my own all morning!" "I'm bloody stuck with the baby all day every day while you're at work," I would counter, and a fight would ensue. Of course we both enjoyed spending quality time with lovely Tori but at the start minding a new baby can be pretty intense and both parents feel it during their respective turns of duty. I remember one evening I was down at the track for Wednesday night racing and I got a phone call after being gone for two hours. It was Cormac. "Please can you come home? She's cutting up rough and I don't know what to do!" "Sure I don't know either!" I countered. "What can I do that you can't?" At this stage I had stopped breast feeding so he couldn't use that as an excuse. I was starting to realise that men, including Cormac, assume women are programmed to look after babies. Maybe we are in a way I suppose. I don't generally like making sexist comments as feel we're all equal in a lot of ways but I think men may actually find the intensity of baby minding harder than women and it wears them down a bit more. Maybe it's something to do with the fact they seem to think they need to do something with the baby when they are minding it, like bathing it, feeding it or bringing it out in the buggy. These seem to be the only options. I know poor Tori got a lot of baths in those early days when I left Cormac on his own with her! Women on the other hand, fit their lives around the baby and could be on the phone, cooking, sending emails or in my case on the rollers all while keeping an eye on the little one.

I did try and be understanding of him and his predicament, but many the power struggle and fight we had during that summer as I tried to get out and Cormac didn't want to be left too long on his own with the baby. Cormac is a very supportive husband and great father but I definitely pushed his limits on more than a few occasions. I think this is probably a feature of my personality. I get extremely zoned in on something and I get somewhat myopic as a result. Poor Cormac would only take so much before he would boil over and I'd have to apologise and row back a bit. Then I'd be pushing the boat out again a week later.

As I said I had to find a way to workout at home. From two weeks post birth, my first priority when Tori went asleep was to jump up on my bike on the rollers and grind out all sorts of workouts. I would be praying she would stay asleep for the required 45 minutes, which in fairness she did a lot of the time. If she was still asleep when I was finished with the rollers, a yoga mat and a medicine ball was a good addition for some core work. On hearing of my rollers exploits, Emma, a sporty friend said to me in exasperation, "I don't know how you manage to get the time – every time I got the turbo and bike set up Eva is awake and crying again!" "Its military precision and focus", I informed her. "You must prioritize the exercise session over everything else! Attention to detail must only be applied to exercise related paraphernalia. The house may be falling down around your ears, the dishwasher may not be emptied, god knows what that thing is living in the drain in the bath preventing the water going out. You just put on those blinkers get up on your bike and get moving! Workout done, hey presto." She laughed. I wasn't joking! "There are unfortunate casualties to this approach of course", I told her "Just ask poor Cormac. He's pretty sick of there being no food in the house and no housework done. In fairness he doesn't expect much and is understanding but does blow up from time to time when things get really bad. Meanwhile I just keep plugging away!" "Your poor husband!", Emma said, genuinely sorry for Cormac, "don't know how he puts up with you!" She was right really, it probably wasn't fair. He just wanted to spend some time with his wife in the evenings, but I was inevitably itching to get out by the time he got home. Then there was the housework issue. I remember one time having an argument about the fact that the kitchen was like an absolute war zone with stuff everywhere. "Someone's got to do a bare minimum of cleaning here to prevent us getting food poisoning", he said in exasperation. "All you think about when the baby goes asleep is training. Then I arrive home and you're gone out the door in the evening again. What do you think you are – an elite athlete?"

Of course I wasn't but when he asked me I realised I was behaving like one. Not that I was at the standard of an elite competitor, but I was treating training as my full time job. And when I wasn't training I was doing that other thing that elite athletes do that is just as important – getting quality rest. I spent an inordinate amount of time that summer watching television with my feet up as I fed Tori and took care of her. The Olympics were on first for two weeks followed by the Paralympics for another two weeks. London 2012 was an amazing show. It was so inspiring. I watched everything from table tennis to shot putt and of course every bit of track cycling that was televised. Watching all these athletes rise and fall in their different disciplines was really amazing. The amount of time and effort that goes into being an athlete at this level was mind boggling. Watching all this glorious competition was probably part of the reason I had no problem staying motivated during the summer after having Tori. I found the track cycling in the Paralympics particularly inspiring. I watched in awe as cyclists missing various body parts rode the 500TT and the Individual Pursuit in a time that would have left me for dead. I was particularly impressed when cyclists were missing one and sometimes even nearly two legs and how fast they could go. There were also a number of Irish competing in the track cycling also which was really great to watch. I particularly enjoyed seeing Catherine Walsh and her pilot Fran Meehan powering around to take the silver medal in the tandem Pursuit. "I would love to pilot one of those bikes someday", I thought. The tandem bikes usually had a visually impaired rider on the back and an able-bodied pilot. I didn't know if I would ever be good enough though as the standard was so high. All the paralympians were now practically training as full time athletes, that was the bare minimum it seemed to be competitive nowadays. That's the beauty of the World Masters I thought to myself– pretty much everyone who rides in it is an amateur and has to hold down a full time job to survive so it's a level playing field. A world championship for ordinary people.

After the Omnium, Hugh encouraged me to get down to the track not just in the evenings but any time there was a session on during the day and bring Tori along. It would certainly solve a lot of problems, I thought to myself. I wouldn't be on the clock for one as there would be no one waiting for me to relieve them of babysitting duties. I hated being on the clock and always felt I was when someone else was minding Tori. On top of that my other option during the day was the rollers and there is only so much of them one can do – my backside couldn't take more than one hour as an absolute max without going into serious protest. Anyone who has ridden rollers will know it can be quite hard on the undercarriage. The weather was also pretty good around that time. "It will be really good for you to get out and not be stuck at home", Hugh suggested when I was procrastinating about bringing the baby, "and good for Tori to, she will get plenty of fresh air. Sure she sleeps half the time anyway so what are you worried about?" "But how will I manage", I protested. "What if she just cries and hates it?" "Why don't you give it a go? And of course you can manage – sure Aidan and Millie practically reared Zach down here last year!" It was true. Aidan and Millie were both into track racing, and had a two year old boy and I saw him frequently at the track. They had a really cool pop up tent that they always brought with them for Zach so he had some shelter if necessary. They used to bring him to the track racing every Wednesday night during the summer and they would take turns racing and minding the baby. The track was ideal for that really and a lot of people brought small children down with them. It's a secure area. When all the riders are in, the gate is locked and no-one else can access the area. The centre of the track is a lovely big green space for people to chill on between training efforts and would be a perfect spot to pitch a tent for the baby. The day after talking to Hugh I went on a shopping trip with Tori and bought a similar tent to the one Aidan and Millie had for Zach – a pretty cheap Gelert pop-up for about €25. The week following the Omnium I rocked up to the track with Tori and the tent for the first time. Prepared for all eventualities I also brought nappies, bottles, toys, rugs and a play mat. On top of all that I also had my bike and gear bag. I realised when I arrived the first day I needed a bloody trailer I had so much gear but made use of Eamonn instead who arrived the same time as me. Eamonn was also being coached by Hugh and was a pretty good sprinter. I still wasn't overly optimistic that bringing the baby was going to work out for me but was determined to try. Hugh was running a special session for me and Eamonn where we were going to work on our 500 TT efforts and our Flying 200s. "This kind of sprint training is perfect for doing with a baby trackside," Hugh had said, "we'll be doing 20-40 second efforts and resting for 5 minutes between each one. So we will be spending more time sitting down on the grass then rolling on the track!" The warm up for a session like that is the only time consuming part, as it takes about half an hour. Tori was in great form and enjoying the trip out and about. I set her up trackside in her car seat and Hugh stayed beside her and ran us through our warm up, where she was happy watching the world and her mom go by every minute or so. At first I was distracted and kept looking but then trusted that all was OK and Hugh would keep an eye on her. Once we had the warm up done and we got down to the various sprint drills to improve our Flying 200's. I transferred Tori to her play mat inside the tent and she played happily with the hanging toys for about half an hour, after which she promptly fell asleep. The session lasted about three hours in total and I was absolutely delighted at the end, in fact I was practically walking on air. I couldn't believe it had worked. I had a new outlet and way to train with a small baby on board. I actually felt the first time was a bit of a fluke and it would never work again. But like the rollers, work it usually did and I wish now I had kept a log of all the times I had her down there in the tent and I got a good session done as I probably wouldn't believe it was possible. I really liked the way I could bring her with me and have her as part of my training session. The very odd day she would start crying but frequently there would be someone trackside to entertain her or pick her up when things got bad and her mom couldn't hear the noise because of the wind in her ears.

I remember one day near the end of the summer when I was doing a short enough training session with Hugh. Tori was at this stage a seasoned visitor to the track and knew the score. We had left her trackside sitting up in her car seat and she was content enough playing with one of her toys while Hugh and I rolled around chatting and warming down after a session. Next thing this lady came up to the fence and started waving at us madly to get our attention. We cycled over. "Is that your baby there", she enquired, pointing at Tori, who at this stage in our lap was on the opposite side of the track to us. I looked at Hugh and him at me. "Yea", I said a bit surprised, and she went along on her way, probably disgusted at the fact that I wasn't within five meters of the baby at all times. "Whose did she think it was?", I asked Hugh as we looked around – there was no one else anywhere nearby and me, Hugh and Tori were the only three souls locked into the big oblong track cage. We had got to the stage where we took Tori's presence so completely for granted at the track we found it quite funny that someone would think it was strange! As we continued on around the track and back over to the abandoned child, I reflected on the fact I had managed to get a good number of sessions in with Tori and done some really good quality training to boot. "I'm so grateful to you for encouraging me" I told Hugh, "If you hadn't suggested I bring her down here it wouldn't have happened. I never thought it would be possible to get good quality training sessions done with a baby on board". "It's easy for me," he said, "You're the one who's doing the work. And I don't mind helping out the odd time as long as when it rains I can share her tent!" I laughed. This had happened once or twice – the heavens had opened up during a session and whoever the first two or three lucky riders were to get to the tent after me would get space to shelter from the rain. Tori thought this was great fun all together, everyone suddenly piling into her tent. Of course she thought we were doing it solely for her amusement.

As the weeks ticked by after the Omnium I got back into a proper training routine, or as proper as one can while minding a baby and the associated restrictions. Looking back, I really did manage to make the best possible use of the time available to me for training during the summer months. Of course, I was limited in what I could do while minding Tori but I continued to exploit my windows. Apparently, one of my top skills according to Cormac – an ability to spot a window where no one else could see one and make use of it. Between sessions on the rollers at home as Tori slept, training at the track in the evenings when Cormac came home, going to the track with Tori during the day and getting out for a few long spins whenever possible I was doing fine. It wasn't optimal but it was the best I could do with my time. However, on the flip side, even though there were time constrains that interfere with training when you have to mind a baby, there are some benefits to these constraints too. You have to train smart. You can't waste time on junk miles. Every session has to count and so on. Another important benefit I believe is that you are forced to rest. Being on maternity leave as a mom minding one baby, you get to hang out a lot. Sitting around, resting those legs between training sessions, allowing them to recover. The biggest stress in your day is trying to figure out where to go for coffee or what to have for dinner. Minding a small baby is really a pretty easy-going existence really once you learn to deal with the mental intensity of it. Especially when you're not given to spending all your free time doing housework. The normal stresses of work do not exist either, which is really good for the body and mind, all of which aids post-exercise recovery. So quality rest and lack of stress are a natural occurrence in your day. I may have been pretty sleep deprived during the summer but at least I was well rested. I had broken sleep and not enough of it but by going to bed early trying to catch up I was lying in a horizontal position for eight to ten hours most nights. Rest is something that most athletes, from elite to weekend warrior alike, don't get enough of. People tend to forget the number one rule of training adaptation – getting fitter, faster and stronger only happens when you rest – not when you train or race. Training just damages your muscles which provides the necessary training stimulus, but if you don't give your body the chance to repair the damage your training has inflicted, you won't get fitter, faster or stronger.

The next event on the calendar for me was the Team Nationals, scheduled to take place at the beginning of August, a few weeks after the Omnium. Hugh wanted Sundrive to make their mark, especially in the sprint events. "I want to get you and Sarah to ride the Team Sprint", he informed us at one of the training sessions. The Team Sprint consists of two people riding a lap as fast as they can from a standing start. The first person leads out and gives everything to their start and pulls up after half a lap. The second person rides in the slipstream of their teammate then gives it their all to take it home when their teammate pulls up. Sarah was one of the few other girls in the club and happened to be a very good starter. My job was going to be to take it to the finish once we got up to speed. This event is very technical and time can be lost as much on getting the technical aspects wrong as not having the speed. Over the few weeks before the event Hugh had Sarah and I repeatedly practice our starts and the changeovers. The hardest thing to get right was the bit where I was to take over from Sarah. The idea was that as we approached the changeover, I had to lie off her rear wheel and at the half lap mark rush into the back of her slipstream, or "the pocket" as it's known, just before she pulled up the track. If this is done correctly it has a slingshot effect and catapults the rider forwards. Sarah had to pull up before a certain point and our wheels couldn't overlap before this or we wold risk disqualification and it was quite hard to get the timing right. I tried the rushing part over and over again. I got the hang of it eventually but there was definitely room for improvement. I wasn't feeling the slingshot effect as much as I should have been. However, given the time we had to practice, Hugh was pretty happy with us as we were posting times of around 40 seconds and weren't likely to get disqualified for passing at the wrong point which was the important thing. It was for this mistake Victoria Pendleton and her GB teammate were disqualified during the Team Sprint in the 2012 Olympics and it cost them the gold medal. "Just a bit more work and I think you girls are in line for a shot at the national title", he told us on one of our training sessions. Myself and Sarah looked at each other, giddy at the thoughts of it. Hugh wasn't given to talking about winning but really felt that the title was there for the taking this year. "Of course it all depends who turns up on the day", he warned, "But I really want you girls to give it your best shot, and if that's good enough, all the better". "You know what that means", I said to Sarah in hushed tones as he walked away, "a national jersey! Oh my God I want one of those so much. We have to win!" The thought of it thrilled her too and gave us an extra kick and more of a focus for our last effort that evening, and we posted our best pre-competition time, 39.89 seconds.

As well as the training for the Team Sprint, we were also training for the Team Pursuit with our Sundrive teammate Caroline, which was being run as a demonstration event on the same day. The men were also putting in a few teams so there were plenty of people down at the team training sessions which were a lot of fun. They took place on Friday evenings. It was training with a social aspect and I was enjoying that as much as anything. People were on wind down after the week and were all pretty relaxed. Eoin Mullen also came along to some of the sessions to practice for the team sprint. It was an added bonus to get to train with him and watch him ride. Eoin is the most promising sprint track cyclist in Ireland and is hoping to ride in the Olympics in Rio in 2016 – I don't doubt he will get there and make his mark. He has the air of a true champion. Eoin is from the Aran Islands off the west coast in Ireland and is an extremely talented young rider. I remember the first time I saw him in action. "Wow", I said in awe to Hugh as he blasted past me at full speed during a team sprint practice, "he looks like he will break the bike in two he's so powerful". "I know" said Hugh, "he was like that the first day he came to the track. I knew the minute I saw him he was something special." I remember watching him practicing rushing at his teammate Donal wishing I could achieve the same effect. Time and time again he was getting into the pocket as he timed it perfectly and visibly accelerated off Donal's wheel.

Eoin was a lovely guy to, really unassuming and easy to chat to as we rolled around warming up. It was great to get out and meet people again and not have baby topics as the main focus of conversation. I wasn't defined as a new mom. On the first nights training one of the guys asked me what I had been up to so far for the summer. When I mentioned having a baby by C-section seven weeks before he was shocked. "My wife didn't get off the couch for three months after she had a baby", he said, "Wait till I tell her about you!" "Yea, that will go down really well", I said, "Just what she needs to hear. Are you mad? She will either feel crap about herself or she will send out a lynching mob to get me for making her look bad!" I had mixed reactions from women when they saw what I was at. Some were so supportive and genuinely amazed I was back competing so quickly. Others I could tell were not so impressed and felt like I was showing them up by my "over-achieving".

Around this time a journalist from the Irish Independent got wind of what I was up to and thought it would make a great story for their supplement, the FIT magazine. She came along to interview me one of the days at the track and had a photographer take pictures of me on my bike and with Tori. The article came out the following week and although, naturally, made me cringe at points, was pretty good. I suppose its normal to be embarrassed when reading about oneself. The title for instance made me squirm a bit: "I cycled 50k on my due date and won a medal six weeks after giving birth". To me it read a bit like "Aliens abducted me and took one of my kidneys"! Overall, the article was generally very well-received but there were a few negative comments from women on Facebook about it. I remember one in particular: "That's all we need – another reason to make us feel bad about our bodies when we are pregnant". That made me feel sad. I felt like this girl had missed the point of the article. Yes, it was about someone who engaged in a lot of physical activity when pregnant and after the birth and this definitely stood to me in many ways in terms of my health, body shape and fitness. And, yes, my article said it was possible to do lots of training when pregnant and have a normal baby at the end. But, more importantly, it was a story about maintaining your identity throughout the whole process. Being fit and competing is a huge part of who I am and I didn't want to lose that aspect of my personality. Many other people would have something different that they would like to keep going throughout pregnancy and motherhood, something that defines them. It doesn't have to be exercise like it was for me. So many women are having babies at a later stage in life now, the average age in Ireland is 31 for first time moms. At this stage people usually have developed lots of interests. It can be a challenge to keep hobbies and stuff going once you get pregnant and have a baby, but my story showed with a bit of effort and help, you can keep whatever your passion in life is up and running, be that crochet or cricket. I wanted other girls to read about me and see there was more to life after baby then nappies and bottles, if they wanted it that is. It's important to specify that. Everyone is different. Some people don't want to keep elements of their pre-baby life, it's as if they enter a new state of mind and everything changes. I remember Hugh saying to me at one stage that I might just want to give up the bike after I had the baby. He warned me that it was possible that I wouldn't be interested in it anymore, or might want to do less of it and not compete. I acknowledged this at the time, even though I couldn't imagine it, I knew it was a possibility.

I remember meeting a girl in my antenatal class about a month before having Tori and she was doing loads of exercise too – pretty physical yoga, swimming and jogging. We had a great conversation about the benefits of exercise during pregnancy and how important it was to us. Three and a half weeks after having Tori I was in the local health centre at a midwives clinic to get her weighed and I bumped into her again. She had had her baby the same time as I. We chatted about how hard it was getting used to the sleep deprivation, feeding issues and so on. Then I asked her whether she had returned to exercise yet. I had just been back on the bike about a week at this point and was a new person for it, expecting she would be somewhat similar. "No", she said staring off into space with that sleep deprived look exclusive to new moms, "I haven't even thought about exercise to be honest. Your priorities just totally change, don't they?" "Hmm, indeed", I responded non-committally. I was so surprised. My priorities had changed alright, I had become even more focussed than ever before on my cycling. Was I a bad mother? I thought I had met a kindred spirit but realised she had completely gone the other way. It was then I realised that everyone truly is different and accepted it. What's right for one may be wrong for another.

As I mentioned earlier, on these club nights Sarah and I were also training with Caroline for the women's Team Pursuit. I absolutely loved this. I had enjoyed the Pursuit so much in the Omnium it was fun to start doing some targeted training for it. Hugh had us doing four lap efforts as fast as we could. It was the first time I had trained properly with pursuit bars and tried to steer the bike with my elbows, which was required when making the changes in the bends during the Team Pursuit. I had tried the pursuit bars during the Omnium and they had been fine, but with the Team Pursuit the rider at the front keeps changing so every few laps you have to be able to steer sharply up the banking and drop back onto the wheel of the second rider precisely coming out of the bend. It was so much fun when we got these changes right. The three of us were like a well-oiled machine and were held up to the boys as the way to do it. We mightn't have been the fastest team there at training but we certainly looked the best. I felt I was definitely getting stronger at the Pursuit during these sessions and my lap times for the four lap efforts were constantly improving. Unfortunately, we didn't have much time as I would have liked to practice, and the day of the Team Nationals rolled around all too quickly.

The main focus of course still was the Team Sprint for me and Sarah, as the Pursuit was only a demo event. There was something really nice about riding with Sarah, it definitely took a bit of the pressure off when compared with an individual event. Of course there was a different sort of pressure on me to perform my best, so as not to let her down, but I didn't feel that would be a problem and was looking forward to the day.

The sun was splitting the stones and there had been a good turnout for the ladies Team Sprint – we had eight teams from all over the country. It was great to see so many. Women's track events in Ireland can really suffer due to lack of riders and often national events get scrapped or demoted to demo events due to lack of numbers. The men's Team Sprint was first so we got to watch Eoin, Donal and another Sundrive rider Keith strut their stuff and annihilate the rest of the field. These guys were so fast and powerful, they were really in a different league, especially Eoin.

Sarah and I warmed up on our turbos side by side in the sunshine and it felt like a perfect day. Hugh had given us a prescribed warm up that lasted 50 minutes, like he does for most events. I loved this as once you start the warm up the butterflies generally disappear and you get to focus on the process. It's like the ball is finally rolling and you just have to get on with it. As the intensity of the warm up increased so did our temperature - we were both nearly melting it was such a warm day. "That's it", I said panting and having enough of being slowly cooked, "it's off with this bloody skin suit, don't care how strange I look in my bra!". I pulled the top half down and it was a relief to feel the breeze on my skin. At least I had a decent black sports bra on and hadn't worn my old washed out grey one! Sarah laughed at me. She had been clever enough to bring a nice skimpy vest for the purpose so didn't have to expose herself No one paid any attention to me as it turned out. We were to ride seventh, the second last team to go. We went off for a last nervous toilet break just before the women started then got back up on the turbos to keep our legs ticking over. Murt, Sarah's boyfriend was there and was really encouraging, clearly he believed in us like Hugh did.

Finally it was our turn. No team had broken 40 seconds yet so I knew if all went smoothly we'd at least get a podium finish. We were held for the start by two burly men. Then the countdown. I was sick with adrenalin. 5..4..3..2..1..GO! Sarah and myself powered down on the pedals and gave it all we had for a great start. We lost a tiny bit of time as we sat down in the saddle but then I timed my rush really well and accelerated off Sarah's wheel at the halfway mark. I rode my heart out for the second half of the lap and literally threw my bike across the line. I listened for the time. "A new fastest time for Sarah and Susie from Sundrive, 39.04". I was delighted! A personal best for us by nearly a second. On the track a second counts for approximately ten bike lengths so that's a pretty good improvement. I came around and dismounted and hugged Sarah. We were both afraid to say anything. We watched nervously as last to go, the the two girls from Orwell, Aideen and Sandy, got ready to start. They were the only thing between us and a national title. We watched and I think I held my breath for the whole lap. "That looked fast" Sarah said as Aideen whizzed over the finish line. Then the time was announced. "39.37", was all I heard. "OH MY GOD Sarah, we've got it!" The two of us hugged again and celebrated. Then I proceeded to hug anyone I could find from Sundrive and beyond as did Sarah. We were so delighted. We both fell upon Hugh, who had gone quiet, as he usually did when he was in shock. He was really pleased for us. It meant we had dominated the sprint events, the two Sundrive teams were national champions. As we warmed down Sarah was really enjoying the sensation. "Yeah, National Champion jerseys, can't believe it", she grinned. "We're so cool! I love this feeling". It had been worth all the effort. She had had some major problems getting time off work for the Nationals but had pulled it off in the end so it was all the sweeter.

Aideen from Orwell, came up to me afterwards to congratulate me. "Another National medal, you're doing so well and just two months after having your baby!" I was a bit embarrassed with all the praise, especially since we had beaten her team into second. What do you say? "Well done to you too, sure you've won loads of national medals now, another one for the collection!", I offered. "But I don't have a national title she said wistfully, that's some achievement – enjoy it", and she walked away. "Another box ticked for you", Hugh said to us later as we finished warming down. "You're national champions now. Most people go all their lives not winning one of those titles. It might never happen again, and it was there for the taking this year. What I'd really like is for you girls to come back next year and break the national record. I think ye can do it, you're less than a second off it!" I was so happy. "If I never win another medal" I thought, "this summer has been great". Two national medals in the bag and one of them a title. Really, I thought things couldn't get any better.

Later on that day we had the Team Pursuit. During training I had showed myself to be the strongest of the three so I was to do an extra lap at the end. I was still so high after the sprint I think I had extra wings. I had the girls ride on their limit whenever I was in front. I was really enjoying it, and we were riding in perfect formation. When I took the front with a lap to go I wound it up as Hugh had told me to do.

Unfortunately, I was so busy winding it up I didn't notice I had lost the two of them off the back of my wheel. It was too late when I saw them and I tried to slow down a bit, but it didn't work. "Whoops", I thought as I crossed the finish line about 100 meters ahead of them, "that wasn't very cool." I was upset I had made a bit of a mess of it at the end as we had perfected a lovely finish in training and our technique had always been about going out to look good riding as a team. I apologised to the girls afterwards for getting carried away. As it turned out we were good enough for silver so that was a nice surprise!

The final event of the day was the Keirin. I loved this race, even though I was pretty new to it. Keirin originated in Japan and the translation of the word is "racing wheels". There is a huge multi-million betting industry build around Keirin racing in Japan. A Keirin usually consists of a few heats and the top riders from each heat go through to a final to battle it out. The race is 2 km long and there are usually six to seven riders in a heat. A derny or motorbike paces the first few laps. The derny starts at 25km/hr and winds the pace up slowly to 45km/hr when it pulls off with 700m to go. The riders have to line up behind the derny which usually involves a lot of jostling and nudging at the start of the race as position behind the motorbike is so important, depending on the rider's strategy. When the durney pulls off after winding up the pace it's a battle for the line. Tactics are very important in Keirin riding and everything from your position behind the derny to timing your jump can be important for success. It can be quite physical too if it comes down to a bunch sprint and there are frequently accidents during the racing. All this makes it a really exciting event to watch.

I rode the first heat and came second so secured my place in the final. Hugh came over to me as I was spinning my legs warming down on the turbo. "I think you should go up a gear", he said. "You'll need to do something different here to win this and a bigger gear will help you go faster. You should play to your strength, go early and go hard". This was all great in theory, but unfortunately the reality didn't quite pan out like that. I think looking back that I was pretty tired and burned out after the two team events. I had also lost my edge to win as I had the national title in my back pocket and couldn't stop thinking about that. Up a gear I went but during the final I got boxed in so didn't get a chance to jump where I had planned. I tried to go a bit later but didn't have the legs to do it dramatically enough and the others just sat on my wheel and came around me at the end before the finish line. I ended up with bronze which I was pretty pleased with but it was bittersweet. "If I had been a bit more focussed I could have won that", I said to Hugh afterwards. "Maybe" he said, "but keirin riding takes a lot of practice to get good at so don't be too hard on yourself. There's always next year, where it will be a full championship event and you have a crack at it then after some more focussed training".

As the day drew to an end Cormac brought Tori to collect me and it was so lovely to see her after all my efforts, it was just the icing on the cake of a great day. I was going around holding her in my arms attracting baby admirers as I went. It was really nice – I found people generally really look at you with a new kind of respect when they see how small your baby is and that you're out there competing, giving it a shot. All in all it turned out to be a pretty good day. One national title and two demo medals and I believed an eight week old beautiful baby to thank for it. Now things definitely couldn't get any better. Or so I thought.

TRAINING-LIFE BALANCE

The following week my mum came up to Dublin on a Tuesday morning to let me out for a training spin. I loved her for this. She would do it every few weeks and I would usually hook up with a friend of mine, Owen, Hugh or whoever was free. She would of course have preferred if I stayed and hung out with her and Tori and drank coffee, but she understood how important getting these spins in was for my training and for my head so she put up with it. That Tuesday Hugh happened to be on a day off so we met up and went for an easy spin and stopped for a coffee half way through. After reflecting on all the achievements to date it was time to move on and focus on the future. "I know I have always been kind of putting you off the Pursuit. It's probably because I felt it's not fun and training should always be fun. But I can't ignore the fact any longer that you are showing real promise at this. I have been watching you come on over the last few weeks starting with that pretty impressive ride in the Omnium so soon after the baby to the few weeks training with the girls for the team pursuit. You're really strong, and getting stronger. I don't see any limits. I think the fact that we have been focussing on sprint training and the 500s has really helped you with the Pursuit. I'm not going to give up trying to turn you into a sprinter but believe you can do both!" I agreed with Hugh. The funny thing was despite that awful first experience in the Nationals in 2011, it had been the first thing that had attracted me to the track, watching the Pursuit on the TV in the 2008 Olympics. I wondered how good I could get.

At that time the autumn track league was also in full swing and Hugh started a plan for the racing for me. On Wednesday evenings racing took place at the track from 6.30pm onwards. The racing was great but it took up the whole evening, most of which was spent hanging around talking. You probably had 20 minutes of track time, depending on the events you were competing in. After one or two nights there and a very irate husband I had to tell Hugh over coffee on that Tuesday spin that the Wednesdays were not an option for me. Cormac was going stir crazy stuck at home with the baby all evening and it wasn't fair on him – I got out enough. It turned out my poor husband, who went to lengths to support me, did have a breaking point. "I understand", Hugh said as he thought about it. "It's important you get some racing experience to sharpen you up though. Tell you what, we can kill two birds with the one stone. Get down to the track Wednesday an hour early and we will take it from there".

The following evening I arrived down early to see what Hugh had in store. "Right", he said. "We're going to ride four lap efforts". Hugh explained that this was the way to train for the Pursuit, shorter efforts then the actual race. Four laps was about 2 km, the Pursuit in the nationals would be 3km. The reason for this was that you could ride these shorter intervals at a higher speed and cadence, and on the day adrenaline would carry you the extra distance, or so one hoped. "I am going to pace you for the first two laps. I will try ride two steady 38 second laps with you in my slipstream and I want you to continue for two more at this pace". We usually did four of these intervals, with breaks in between. It was a really good tough session and became a regular pre-race fixture for me on a Wednesday evening. Sean, my Sundrive teammate who was also training for the Pursuit nationals, frequently joined me on these Wednesday slots and we would ride together and discuss pacing strategy, aerodynamics and all sorts of stuff and generally have a laugh. On these Wednesdays I would also hang around and do the first race or two of the league as well so would get a little racing experience. This meant I was able to get home to Cormac within two hours – a nice window as I arrived back before the novelty of minding the baby wore off. It also meant the evening wasn't gone and we had some time to spend together. With me training so much and my tendency to run out the door as soon as he arrived our relationship was suffering a bit and it was hard to get to spend any decent time together. The fact that we were both wrecked from baby induced broken sleep meant bedtime was now frequently 9.30pm or even earlier didn't help. Of course we got to spend time together with the baby but I found that when she was awake, the focus was very much on her. Also the conversations tend to revolve around baby-related topics. "Did you change her nappy before you put her in bed? How much of that bottle did she drink?" Sometimes too it was hard not to take these statements personally. "Of course I changed her nappy before putting her to bed", I'd snap back. Cormac would generally feign innocence and claim to have meant nothing by the question but I had a bit of a chip about it I suppose. It's amazing, but the arrival of a new baby totally takes the focus off your own relationship, which is not a good thing, and I can totally understand the need to actively make time for your partner when a new baby comes on the scene, or it can take its toll. I think during this time I was also a bit paranoid about my baby-minding, and thought Cormac felt I shouldn't be spending so much time training and more with baby. He claims that this was all in my head so will give him the benefit of the doubt!

Around this time too, I was in communication with my boss from work. I had given him a call to see how he was getting on and how things were going. I had kind of turned a blind eye to work even though I thought I would be chomping at the bit to get back within a few weeks of having the baby. Maybe I would have had I not been so focussed on the bike. Turned out he was in a bad way. Things were going pretty badly for the fish industry. It was the summer from hell. There was a gill parasite, an amoeba that was wreaking havoc for the entire salmon farming industry in both Ireland and Scotland. It was causing a disease called amoebic gill disease, or AGD for short, and was having a terrible impact on some sites in terms of mortality and growth. To top this off I discovered the American girl my boss had hired to replace me while on maternity leave wasn't allowed to work as a vet in Ireland despite the fact that she had been granted a visa. The Veterinary Council had made a decision not to accredit her qualification as she was American, even though she had done her veterinary degree in Edinburgh University in Scotland. A Scottish person or even a European who had received their degree there would not have been a problem. We had gone to so much trouble to get her a visa, having to prove there was no Irish or even European vet that would or could do the job (we advertised but not a single Irish vet showed any interest). To rub salt in the wound she had returned to Scotland and got a job with our main competitor. Hamish was a bit put out to say the least. Not to mention trying to do the work of three people on his own. With all this going on poor Hamish must have been under severe stress. It was a major wake up call for him. He no longer had me to rely on and I felt bad about that, even though there was nothing I could do. I decided that now would not be the time to share the news of how I was doing so well on the bike. Better he thought I was housebound chained to the baby.

It really made me realise though how lucky I was with the timing of the birth. Even though it was bad timing for the maternity leave from a work point of view, it was great for me in terms of the track. My workload is usually substantial during the summer months as that's when fish develop all sorts of health problems. I said a silent thank you to all those who had delivered this baby to me at the start of the summer and given me a break from work during this period. There's no way I could do my job full time and do even half the training I was getting done on maternity leave. Not to mention my job is pretty physical and when I'm not jumping on and off boats and hauling nets and hefting fish around I'm driving hundreds of miles. In my experience, I don't know why but driving can be as tiring for the legs as doing something strenuous. So I decided I had to make the most of this summer as this kind of freedom might never happen again. As Cormac was at pains to remind me, with good reason, even though I was "rimming it" with all the training I was doing, I wasn't a full-time athlete. Well I knew that being on maternity leave was probably the closest I was going to get and I vowed to make the most of it.

I had promised Hamish I would come back in November, when Tori was five months old. I felt that this was a good compromise on my part. Tori wouldn't be so young going to the crèche, and I wouldn't be taking the full time allowed on maternity leave. I won't lie, another reason I left it until November was that I wanted to get to the Worlds in good shape without the stresses of work impinging on me and with plenty of time to rest beforehand when I was tapering the training. Always an ulterior motive.

In the weeks between the Team Nationals and the National Champs, on top of the pursuit sessions, I was doing the occasional sprint training session with Eamonn and Hugo, two other riders Hugh was coaching. The four of us would practice our starts and do short intense sprint efforts. We also spent time practicing some match sprinting, which I was pretty awful at. I seemed to suffer from brain freeze when forced to make tactical decisions. Hugh assured me that this would come with practice, but I wasn't so sure. I knew I had the engine, and reasonable speed, just sometimes I wasn't so sure about my operating system. These sprint-training sessions involved a lot of short intense efforts and we would rest between them to allow the body time to recover. The sessions were fun, lounging about on the grass having a laugh with the lads. Tori was frequently present as many of the sessions took place during the day when the lads were off work and she provided a bit of distraction for everyone there. She was becoming more and more interactive with each passing day. She loved Eamonn in particular and always beamed when she saw him. "It's the bald head Susie", he informed me rubbing his shaved crown, "she recognises a kindred spirit!" On top of one of these sessions a week, I was trying to do intervals on my rollers twice a week. I was doing four minute efforts, usually about four to six of them trying to recreate the feeling of the Pursuit. For these efforts, I focussed more on leg speed rather than pushing a big gear. I wanted my legs to get used to spinning at the high cadence of 120rpm for the four minute duration required during the Pursuit. I figured I wasn't achieving this sort of cadence in practice but was maybe managing about 100 - 110. Cadence sessions were good to do on the rollers when Tori was sleeping, as from start to finish only took about 50 minutes.

The week before the Nationals Hugh put me on a serious taper. I was basically to do nothing, just one or two easy sessions near the start of the week, nothing on Wednesday or Thursday and very light rollers for about 20 minutes on Friday, the day before the event. Eoin was at the track training session on the Monday and I asked him what he would be doing that week as I really thought Hugh was telling me to do too little. "Yea, I won't be doing much, just the rollers for maybe twenty minutes, half an hour on Friday with two or three sprint efforts to wake up the muscles." Good enough for Eoin Mullen was good enough for me and I decided I should trust Hugh's plan, even though the concept of tapering was alien to me. It was an awful week I remember – like being on cold turkey from alcohol or drugs. My body was clearly addicted to exercise and it couldn't understand what was going on all of a sudden. In protest, my legs started to feel really achey and I was getting twinges in my knee and one of my hips and my quads started to feel really heavy, like I had done loads of training. But Hugh remained adamant I had to do as little as possible. "My legs feel awful!" I wailed to Eamonn on the phone. "I'm the same Susie", he informed me, having been put on a similar regime. "I've developed pains where I never had injuries and my calves feel like cement!" The fact he was suffering too made me feel slightly better. "You've just got to trust me on this one", Hugh said, when I whined to him that I felt I was losing my fitness. "This is a minor taper. You'll be on a much longer one prior to the Worlds next month". I was horrified!

"Look", he reassured me, "you've done all the work, you've done the training. Just trust your body. You have never ever underperformed on the day since I have known you. You always raise your game for the big occasions. The weekend will be no different. We're just looking to post some really good times, this is more part of your training for the worlds, there will be no pressure on you to win medals. I reckon you're capable of a 4.22 or so in the Pursuit. Looking at the entry list it's hard to say but riding a time like that would put you about fifth. That's all we want. It will be a good experience and show your training is on track for the worlds. And the last thing we want is you bursting yourself and riding a time that puts you fourth and into the bronze medal ride off. A ride off you probably won't win which will just exhaust you as you'll have to do two Pursuits on Saturday and that would just mess up your chances in the sprinting!" I relaxed a bit but my legs still felt awful. The tapering messes with your head as well as your body as you start to doubt yourself as it gives you way too much time to think. I didn't sleep very well on the Friday night and was so glad when the Saturday dawned, nice, fresh and sunny.

It was always great to be down at the track in this kind of weather. I got down early and got set up and started my warm up. The Women's Pursuit was the second event so there was plenty of time to get setup. Hugh wasn't there as he had been asked to do the cycling commentary for the London Paralympics, so I had young Hugo as my assistant instead. Hugh had asked him to take care of me and he was making a good job of it, which was sweet. Hugo was 17 but looked like he was well into his 20s or even 30s due to his muscular build and ability to produce facial hair far beyond his years. He had just taken up the track that summer and had great aspirations to ride for Ireland someday in the sprint events. He was showing a lot of promise for someone who had just started and Hugh had high hopes for him. He was running about offering me drinks, checking my bike, changing gears for me and so on. As I rolled around during the warm up I chatted to Greg, an American cyclist who had been living in Ireland for many years. He had a lovely drawly American accent, which I found relaxing to listen to. He was primarily a road rider but liked to dabble in the Pursuit on the track and I had met him at the Masters the previous year. "Any tips Greg?", I asked. He looked me up and down. "Borrow an aero helmet. Get some shoe covers. And ditch those gloves!" I could borrow a helmet and shoe covers off my teammate Caroline. "Are you serious about the gloves?" I asked having never considered riding without them. "Hell yea", he said, "they create drag. Every split second counts here girl". I took all his advice, just in case.

Before long it was time. I was scheduled to ride against Geraldine Gill in the second pairing. She was a good rider, having been National Road Race Champion on several occasions in the past. Hugo had accompanied me to the start. "Now I'll call out your lap times just beyond the pursuit line", he informed me pointing to where he would stand. "Don't go out too hard!" he warned sternly. He was taking his job seriously. I was totally hyped on adrenaline as I really wanted to post a good time in this event, which I had developed a secret love for. I didn't know why I loved it so much as it was so bloody hard. Maybe that's why I did love it though. People always say there's nowhere to hide in the Pursuit. It's just the rider at his or her limit trying desperately to judge a measured effort so they don't burn up and fade out, or worse still finish with something in the tank. Anyway at the gun I put the foot down and despite my intentions went out way too hard. I realised this as I blasted past Hugo after one lap and he shouted 36! "Jesus", I thought, "I better take the foot off the gas or I will die". I eased off ever so slightly but didn't want Geraldine to get ahead of me either so was conscious of that. "37" Hugo shouted, I could just about hear him as the wind whistled past the aero helmet I had borrowed from Caroline, my Sundrive teammate. "37" he roared again, 37"...more wind, "38" my legs were starting to tire as I struggled to ignore the burning sensation. "37" I heard the bell signifying the last lap, just buried myself and focussed on the line and finally made it across the finish. With that I nearly passed out. I was panting hard as I half rolled, half staggered over to the fence where I collapsed leaning against it and could hardly unclip my feet. I dismounted and collapsed face down on the grass. Hugo was standing over me. "Great ride!" he said, "you did 4.18! You beat Geraldine by a second!" I was absolutely thrilled. "Now help me up!" I couldn't believe how good my time was. I would have been happy with a figure in the low twenties but had knocked a whopping 12 seconds off my time since the Omnium six weeks previously.

I had no idea what would happen next but as I watched the others whom I expected to beat me ride one after another they didn't. Next thing I knew it was down to the final pairing, both of whom were elite riders and shoe-ins for the gold medal ride off. Oh God, I said to Sean, as realisation dawned, "I'm in the bronze medal ride off!" I wasn't sure how I felt about it. It hadn't been part of the plan. And it was totally going to mess up the sprinting. "And what's more", Sean said, "You're going in in third position. You've a really good chance of a medal". He was in exactly the same position as I, having qualified third with a great ride in the men's competition. "But I'm so wrecked after that I told him, I've no chance!" "Don't be silly, she's wrecked to. I saw her, she really started slowing in the last lap. You just got stronger. You can beat her!" We chatted as we rolled our legs on our turbos to warm down. I was so thrilled with myself. I didn't care if it messed up the sprinting. I was within sight of a bronze medal in the Individual Pursuit, a truly special accolade. I wished Hugh had been there to see it. I was on a high. I was feeling a little emotional with some tears threatening too – I was wondering what was wrong with me but realised after a quick calculation it was just before my period so all the feelings were probably exaggerated. I didn't feel in tip top shape physically as a result of being pre-menstrual, I had some mild cramps and water retention, but I realised after my performance in the Pursuit it mustn't have been affecting me. Interestingly, later that week I read in a physiology book that many women perform best at this time of the month, in and around the start of menstruation. Apparently, a woman's VO2 max, or aerobic potential, fluctuates during the monthly cycle and is actually at its peak at this time. So even though you can feel awful and you might even cry, your performance capability is probably enhanced. There are so few benefits of being pre-menstrual, I was glad to have finally found a useful one!

The next event in the Nationals was the Flying 200 to qualify for the sprint rounds. I rode well and I saw the clock stop at 13.99 as I crossed the line and roared "Yeeessssss!", and punched the air. I was delighted as it was my first time to break 14 seconds. A few people were laughing at me and my crazy celebrations. "You'd swear you'd just broken the national record or something", one of the stewards said to me good naturedly as I dismounted. It might not have been quite record-breaking but to me it meant a lot. I felt 14 seconds was one of those pivotal time markers to break, a bit like 40 seconds for the 500TT. Once I had achieved that I felt I could keep chipping away and would hopefully get closer to 13 the following year. The celebrations were short-lived though as it was back on the bike and time to focus on the warm up for the Pursuit bronze medal ride off. I felt pretty strong during the gradual warm up, nervous, excited and relaxed all at the same time. Sean was warming up beside me for his ride off in the men's. "The bronze medal ride off is actually pretty special", he said. Sean loves competition so was eagerly awaiting his turn. I was nervous and more so just wanted to get it over with. "Think about it", he went on. "It's more of a challenge then the gold medal ride – at least the loser there takes home a silver. If you don't come out on top in this one you go home with nothing!" He was right, I realised. The pressure was on to perform and this focussed my mind on the task at hand. Sean won his medal, and then it was my turn to give it a go. I steadied myself in the start gate and went out hard again but took the foot slightly off the gas as I sat down. This time I rode a bit more steadily and my lap times were more consistent and I just wound it up slightly as I got nearer the end. Although I couldn't see Geraldine, Sean was standing at the pursuit line letting me know I was slightly up on her and increasing my lead slightly with every lap. I wasn't even listening to Hugo shouting lap times at me, I was just completely focussed and in the zone. It was over so quickly and next thing I knew I had won comfortably in an even faster time of 4.16. I really couldn't believe it, not only had I won bronze but I had gone faster second time around! What's more, Geraldine had done the opposite and was three seconds slower than me this time. "4.16", I breathed to myself, "I can't believe it". And a beautiful National Medal in the Individual Pursuit to reward my efforts. It felt great to win a medal in this discipline. It's the one every track rider respects due to the nature of it, a true test of fitness and endurance, you try to ride to your limit and leave it all out there on the track. I stood on the podium with Caroline Ryan and Lydia Boylan, two seriously good cyclists who rode at a high level. And there was me, first time mom with only a year on the track. I was indeed in esteemed company.

After the medal presentation I floated about the track on a high, I couldn't focus on anything else. Unsurprisingly, after that I made a mess of the sprinting! Geraldine in fact was matched against me in the Match Sprint and got her revenge by knocking me out. I didn't care. All of a sudden I was being viewed a bit differently by everyone. No longer were people saying well done a great achievement for someone who has just had a baby to me, but they were saying, well done a great achievement in its own right. I had kept up this cycling thing and pursued a dream as I didn't want to lose what defined me when I became pregnant and had a baby. The funny thing was I hadn't lost my identity but had actually found a new one, as a credible athlete. To be viewed as such meant a lot to me.

Cormac was absolutely delighted for me when I got home that evening and recounted the day's events. I had a lovely evening relaxing and recovering and spending some quality time with him and Tori and was completely chilled about day two. I slept like a log that night, and Cormac did both the night feeds to allow me to get in those extra few hours' sleep. The next morning dawned sunny and warm again, it seemed the weather gods were smiling down on Dublin for a change. Again, I got down to the track early allowing myself plenty of time for the warm up. I was really looking forward to the 500TT as we had put a lot of work into this event all summer and I wanted to see if I could significantly improve my time. Looking at the line up I reckoned I had a chance of a medal but wasn't going to get too hung up on that, especially after winning the bronze in the Pursuit. I was scheduled fifth last to go. I got up on my bike in the gate feeling amped and nervous. This event is like that. Hugh had taught me you really had to be 110% switched on and rearing to go as the start was hugely important. I concentrated really hard on the beeps and the countdown..5..4..3..2...1 and on go I launched myself forwards out of the gate with every ounce of aggression I could muster. After this short intense bout of aggression required for the start I concentrated on pedal strokes four through eight, where I have a tendency to slack off a bit, then I switched to concentrating on accelerating as I sat down in the saddle, another place where I sometimes loose time. I pushed as hard as I could and felt my legs starting to die as I rounded the last corner for home. I could see the clock at the end of the straight as I raced towards it. 39..40..I gave a final push as my legs were tying up in a knot from the exertion, trying with everything to get the bike across the line before 41.. It felt like the longest second of my life. 41.1 I crossed the line and the clock stopped. I punched the air again followed by another noisy celebration. I was thrilled with my time as I hadn't recorded anything faster than a 41.8 in training. An improvement of 0.7 of a second, seven bike lengths – it was turning out to be another good day. I was pretty happy with my time as I sat back to watch the other girls go. One after the other they rode slower than me – I couldn't believe it. Finally, it was just Lydia Boylan left, which meant I had a silver medal in the bag! Lydia was a shoe in for the gold as is the fastest female sprinter in Ireland. She rode a great time of 39.4 that day to take the champions jersey leaving me with the silver. Again I was on the podium in esteemed company. "There's something really nice about silver", Hugh said to me afterwards. I agreed, especially when it came so unexpected. The Scratch Race was scheduled for later that day so I relaxed a bit after the 500 and enjoyed the buzz in the track centre, chatting to people and drinking tea. Cormac came down with Tori and we hung out on the grass for a while before it was time to get up and do it all again. There were all sorts of tactics being talked about for the Scratch race among the female riders. We all knew Caroline Ryan and Lydia Boylan would be the two big guns and the other girls were suggesting all sorts of strategies to keep them under control during the race, which went in one ear out the other for me. As we pulled away from the fence it was immediately pretty high octane racing with all sorts of attacks going on and I alternated between chasing people down to hanging onto wheels. While I was going well in the timed events, I'm afraid my brain hadn't really switched onto the finer points and tactics of bunch racing yet, maybe that would come when I had more experience. People are always riding on my wheel and then coming around me at the end. Today was no different and I think I came fifth overall or another equally meaningless position. "God that Scratch race I won in the Omnium was a pure fluke", I reminisced as I rolled for a lap with my tail between my legs. Overall though I wasn't upset. I knew winning the silver that morning had taken the edge of me and I had probably relaxed a little too much prior to the scratch race. I had won national medals in my two favourite disciplines on the track so it had been a pretty special weekend for me all in all. My silver on day two had also cemented people's belief in me as a credible rider, which felt pretty good all told. It was hard to believe how well things had been going for me this summer.

The week after the Nationals I went around in a bit of a daze. The excitement of winning those two medals just didn't seem to be wearing off. I have mentioned how important it was to me that people were actually seeing me as a credible athlete now, but I was also just getting to grips with this myself. I was looking at myself with new eyes, and wondering just how fast I could go. My improvements in the Pursuit had been so astounding it was a bit of a wake-up call. I had gone 14 seconds faster than the Omnium, after just six weeks of training. "How far can I take this?", I asked Hugh. "I don't see any limits", he replied. He had said that to me once before and I was starting to believe him. While I was daydreaming about the possibility he might be right I kept thinking of Keanu Reeves' character "Neo" from the film The Matrix. "He's beginning to believe," were the Oracles words, as he got to grips with the fact he was something special. Being one of my favourite films ever and definitely the one I have watched the most times (10+ at a conservative guess) I think The Matrix is embedded in my subconscious and comes to mind in moments like these! And like Neo, I was beginning to believe too. "It's just unfortunate that time is not on your side", Hugh went on "But we won't let that stop us and we'll see what you can do. I can't believe someone didn't get a hold of you when you were younger, God knows what you could have done. But that's the beauty of the Masters Championships – it's there for you now. You will someday be a Master's Champion, I promise. It mightn't happen this year or next year but you will get there." I reflected on this but couldn't imagine it. It seemed like a pipe dream, so far away. "I think all the specific sprint training we did for the 500s and the Flying 200s may have paid dividends for your Pursuit. It's definitely partly responsible for your improvements. And as the pursuit in the Masters is only 2 km, it will suit you even better. We will do some more specific training for the Pursuit between now and then but also keep up the sprint work".

I read up a bit about this afterwards, and it turned out there was actually good evidence that sprint-type training was effective for the Pursuit. The Pursuit uses a combination of both the bodies' aerobic and anaerobic systems. Estimates suggest its approximately 80% aerobic and 20% anaerobic, so it's essential to have the anaerobic system in tip top shape to optimise your time in this event. There is further evidence to suggest that the balance is tipped even further towards riders with increased anaerobic capacity for a 2 km Pursuit which may even be up to 30% anaerobic. Another advantage of the sprint training was the fact we were always practicing standing starts for the 500TT. Hugh reckoned that people underestimated the importance of the start in the Pursuit and most people don't put enough effort into it, afraid they would pay for it later on. But Hugh believed it was worth an extra kick of effort. "Think about it" he explained to me, "If you do a good fast start you will hit your cruise speed a few seconds before you would with a conservative start." It turned out he was right. We did a session at the track focussing on starts and by the end realised that a little extra effort and the start would mean reaching cruise speed about two seconds earlier then a more moderate start and this obviously had a significant impact on overall time.

During the few weeks after the Nationals I chipped away on my Pursuit. I continued the Wednesday evenings when possible and we added an extra specific training session on a Saturday morning. I loved these Saturday sessions. It was usually just me, Sean and occasionally another very talented road and track rider from Southern Ireland, Hugh Mulhearne. Hugh was a lovely guy and he had ridden a very good Pursuit in the Nationals in 2011, only being beaten by Martyn Irvine, a full-time elite athlete, an Irishman currently competing with great success on the track at international level (At the time of writing Martyn had just won silver at the 2013 World Championships in the Pursuit, and gold in the Scratch Race). Hugh had taken the national title in 2012 when Martyn didn't show up, but I think he would have given him a good run for his money if he had. All three of us, Sean, Hugh and I were going to the Masters in Manchester and targeting the Pursuit as our main event. On these Saturday mornings I would get up at 7am or so have a good feed of porridge and sneak out, all my gear ready to go from the night before. If Tori was awake I'd take her downstairs and give her a bottle for breakfast. Then around 7.45, just before I had to leave, I'd nip upstairs and dump her on top of poor sleeping Cormac, trying my best to give him the maximum lie in. This alleviated my guilty conscience somewhat for leaving him.

The weather always seems to be better in Ireland first thing in the morning for some reason and this turned out to be the case on most of those Saturdays. Although sometimes it was a bit chilly, there was usually no wind or rain to contend with, both of which provide their challenges on an outdoor track. On these mornings we'd do some team pursuit intervals in formation, changing every half lap as part of the warm up and then we would individually take turns doing our efforts. I remember one morning I asked Hugh Mulhearne to act as my derny for a few laps. I knew he was cranking out very fast laps of around 34 – 35 seconds but I thought I might manage to hang on his wheel for one or two of these. "Don't mind me", I said, "you just work away at your effort. I'll be right on your wheel for a few laps then I will pull up when I'm getting tired". That turned out to be a bit of over planning on my part. As Hugh wound up the speed with me on his wheel to make his effort he suddenly launched himself off the banking towards the pursuit line at such speed I completely lost him within about two seconds. I furiously tried to catch up with him for a lap or so but not a chance that I could reel him in. I was a bit embarrassed to say the least. When he asked me enthusiastically afterwards, "How was that?", I realised he hadn't even noticed what had happened, so I replied "Grand, didn't stay with you for as long as I planned but thanks anyway". He was so focussed he hadn't even noticed he had burned me off before he even crossed the start line! During the sessions I would usually manage about four hard three lap efforts. I had shortened the efforts from four to three laps now as the Pursuit in the Masters was 2 km, so my efforts were around 1.5 km, and hopefully on the day I would be able to maintain this speed for the full distance.

In between the training sessions I was really enjoying this month hanging out with Tori. It was coming to the end of my maternity leave and I wanted to make the most of the time I had with her. The shock of being responsible for another individual for the rest of my life had finally worn off, or maybe I had just acclimatised. She was really developing her own little personality and was quite independent and strong minded in ways. "That's right Tori, keep fighting for your rights!", Cormac's mum had commented one evening when Tori was wailing as she had enough of looking at her hanging mobile and wanted out of the cot. That was her all over, fighting for her rights. But overall she was a really sunny baby and always up for a laugh. She didn't startle easily or ever make strange with new people. She loved doing her own thing but liked you to keep it interesting for her and frequently change the record. Kick mat to mobile to sitting in her chair to tummy-time, and a good spin in the buggy to top it all off. Just keep it moving. I found it amazing how such a young small individual could have such a strongly developed personality already. We would frequently have little battles of wills where she might want to be moved from her chair to her kick mat and I'd be determined to finish my last few minutes on the rollers. She would usually win too as would crank up the volume and I didn't want the neighbours ringing social services. It was a really lovely time though and I felt blessed to be able to take the time out to spend with her. And to think I had been worried that I didn't love her as much as I felt I was supposed to at the start. I thought back to a conversation I had with Hugh about three weeks after having Tori. He had agreed to meet me for an easy spin in the park as I hadn't been out on the road with the bike yet. I had something on my mind. "Do you remember when I told you I was pregnant", I asked him, "and you said something to me then that's sort of niggling at me now. You told me the love you have for your children is like nothing else you've ever experienced. Well I don't feel like that and I'm worried something is wrong with me!", I blurted out. To my surprise, he laughed at me, "Don't be ridiculous, of course you love her. I can see by the way you are taking care of her and nurturing her there's huge love there! And it will grow, you have to get to know her first." I smiled remembering how sure he was. Even though I wasn't sure I believed him, his words had made me feel better at the time. Looking back I could see now he was totally right. I think I was still awash with hormones and the shock hadn't worn off so couldn't see it myself. No one really tells you that this is normal though at the time, it's like a taboo subject. I hadn't wanted to say it to Cormac or my mum as they were nearly to close and I didn't want to worry them so I needed some alternative input. Sometimes it's easier to talk to people on the outside and I felt I could say it to Hugh without being judged. In reality, it's when the child's personality comes to the fore that the real parental love does.

Tori and I spent plenty of time out and about going for long walks, relaxing and frequently stopping for coffee. By this stage I was accustomed to bringing her to the track and was pretty relaxed about it so frequently brought her along to daytime training sessions. Around this time I was also up and down to Carlow a bit to visit my parents which was really nice. Tori was now getting more used to travelling in the car. She had been a nightmare at the start, sometimes wailing for up to half an hour, which is a long time to be stuck in a car with a crying baby. When I was in Carlow I'd get a chance to pop out on my bike for a spin and mum was delighted to mind Tori. Tori loved mum and dad too, and I could see why, they were like her servants, always at her beck and call. My mother wouldn't put her down. "She'll expect me to carry her around everywhere now too!" I chided, but I didn't really mind as was delighted Tori was developing such a good relationship with her grandmother. I thought my dad had gone slightly mad, as had never seen him pay so much attention to a baby. I think he must have been worn down by the previous six grandchildren and had no resistance left by the time Tori arrived.

During a visit, I told mum that Cormac wanted me to leave the Masters and go next year instead. Even though she thought I was mad and totally overdoing it with all the training, she knew how much I wanted to compete and gallantly offered to mind Tori for the full duration while I was gone to Manchester. "That would be great mum", I said, as I knew

Cormac was really a bit anxious about being left with her for the week on his own. "That will take the heat off me for running off!" My brother happened to be home from Australia at this time and he also promised to help out. He rang me when mum explained to him I was feeling a bit guilty leaving Cormac in the lurch. "Whatever support is required I will provide", he promised. "It's so brilliant you're doing this going and competing. I wish it was me!" He had always been really into sport too and had a phase of competing seriously in triathlon a few years previously, and was now a pretty committed recreational mountain biker. I was delighted to have his support too.

I had decided to book into the same hotel I had stayed in the previous year for the Masters as I would know what to expect. The Holiday Inn Express in Manchester wasn't too fancy but it ticked all the boxes and the staff was friendly. A few of the others were also staying there including Sean and some of the girls and it would be nice to have people around. I had really been ahead of the game and had booked the room two months in advance. Needless to say I got a bit of a shock when I decided to ring the week before and specify I wanted a quiet room and was informed they had no record of a booking for me. And what was more there was no rooms left in the hotel. I had a day or two of panic but managed to convince them I had room definitely been booked for me and they "double booked" me again. I breathed a sigh of relief, that was one stress I didn't need! It was a lot more hassle then the previous year trying to organise everything with Tori to think of too.

I understood why Cormac was a bit nervous about being left on his own. He was fantastic with Tori and loved her so much and they had a great relationship already. Having said this Cormac was still a man, a father, and their role is different from that of the mother. I hadn't realised that this would be the case so much but it's definitely true what they say: a father might die for his children but a mother lives for them. No matter how good a husband is, most of the day to day hard graft and the caring and nurturing is done by the mother. She puts the hours in. She is the one on maternity leave and that's probably why it's so intense for her at the start. At least the father gets to go back to work after a week or so. Cormac acknowledged that minding Tori could be difficult at times and he mostly let me out training to give me a much needed break, even though I knew he would have liked me to be around a bit more at that time.

All in all, it was a good time. I had no idea how much I was improving or had improved since the Nationals so around two weeks before Manchester Hugh thought it would be a good idea for me to ride the Pursuit in the Veterans Omnium just to get a time to see where I was at. There was a 2 km Pursuit, like the Masters. I rode a 2.49 which was pretty good considering I only had my training wheels on the bike and no aero helmet. I was taking to Terry afterwards as I was wondering how that would relate to an indoor Pursuit of the same distance. "You should able to go five to six seconds faster, Terry reckoned. That would give me a 2.43 I calculated. Not bad, I thought, and based on the times from last year if I could push it a little more. I might even scrape into the bronze medal ride off. Hugh had me on another even stricter taper so it was nice to see that I was improving and not losing my fitness. This is something that is always niggling at the back of everyone's mind when they back off the training. It seemed everything was going according to plan, however, and I was hopeful I would go and give a good account of myself in Manchester.

WORLD CHAMPION

"He makes the clouds his chariot, and rides on the wings of the wind".
Psalm 104

A few days before I was to head off for Manchester I was not feeling the best. I developed a head cold. Yes, I had actual symptoms, dry throat, headache and stuffy nose, but I also believe it was partly in my head. Every athlete's worst nightmare is that they will get sick just before an event. All that build up, all that training, then bang! A flu floors you and performance goes out the window. The hassle of arranging people out to have mind Tori had been getting on top of me and I was starting to wonder if it was worth it. I also wondered if I should be going. I had a few rows with Cormac in the run up to going as it was a major inconvenience to him to mind her even with my mum on board to help. The truth was he really didn't want to be left on his own with her. It would be the first time he would be in such a situation and I think he was quite apprehensive about it all. Trying one last time he begged, "Sue, could you not just leave it this year when she is so young? It will be there for you again next year". This statement came at the end of one of the rows and I have to say I nearly cancelled the trip. I was worn out with the hassle and the fact I wasn't feeling 100% wasn't helping either. With the hotel double booking my room too it just seemed like all was going against me, if I were to believe in omens.

In spite of everything, however, when the Sunday afternoon rolled around, I packed the car and boarded the ferry in Dublin Port for the short crossing. As I drove off the boat at the far side and headed for Manchester guided by my sat-nav, feeling all heady, I did wonder again whether Cormac was right. Maybe I should have left it. "Why am I doing this?" I asked myself. My headache was worsening and I felt I really needed to take something for it. I texted my friend Una who works for the anti-doping unit of the Irish Sports Council. On the off chance I was going to get drug tested I wanted to be sure I didn't take anything questionable. She assured me regular paracetamol or ibuprofen was fine. I drove straight into the nearest ASDA and bought some of both. Thankfully things started looking up when I arrived at the hotel. The paracetamol was kicking in and some of the Irish crew were there already hanging in the lobby – Tonya, Orla and Sean and talking to them I started to get excited. With all the logistics I hadn't had time to think until then about the fact that I was going to be competing in the World Masters. A shiver of anticipation ran through me. I slept pretty badly that night. It was my first time away from Tori and I kept waking up. I felt somewhat cheated as I thought I would get a magnificent night's sleep once I was away from her looking for her 3am feed.

The following morning I woke with a blinding headache again and was feeling a bit woozy when I staggered out of the bed. I switched to the ibuprofen and had breakfast. After a few cups of tea I felt a bit better and headed down to the track to set up all my gear. I always get a thrill of excitement when I walk into the centre of a velodrome. As you come up into the track centre, there's something awesome about it all. The beautiful symmetry of the structure and those sheer walls of shiny wood just makes me catch my breath every time no matter where I am. I got a few butterflies and set up my rollers for 20 minutes of easy spinning to knock the travel out of my legs. Even though my head felt awful my legs felt pretty good so I was happy about that. I hung out with the guys and soaked in the atmosphere a bit, had a bite of lunch and then headed back to the hotel to relax for the afternoon. I was starting to get pretty excited. That strange mix of dread and anticipation was kicking in. The women's 500TT was on in the evening session but we weren't sure what time. I went down early to be sure I had plenty of time to do a structured warm up. I had a set protocol to follow that Hugh had given me which took about 90 minutes. Once I started that process the inevitable countdown to the event would be underway and the waiting around over. I was determined to go well in this. Last year I got stuck in the gate and had done a relatively poor time. I really wanted to break 40 seconds this year. The best I had done was a 40.8 and that was on the outdoor track at Sundrive. I thought I could surely go a second faster indoors without the wind and other external factors to contend with. Before I knew it, I was in the gate watching the clock counting down. I was concentrating really hard on doing the perfect start. Beep! 10 seconds to go. Settle into the handlebars, looking straight ahead. Beep! 5 seconds. Deep breath. Beep! 4. Beep! 3. Beep! 2. Stand up. Beep! 1 second. Lean back...and GO! I went as hard as I could out of the gate stomping my foot down on the left pedal. I felt like I was going well but lost a bit of speed going around the first bend as the bike was all over the place and I also slowed slightly when I sat down and settled into the bars. I pushed hard, crossed the line and looked at the clock –it stopped at 40.04 – I was so disappointed! I had missed my target by 4/100 of a second. It was a reasonable time but I just had wanted to break the 40 mark so much. However I had to put that aside and move on, there was nothing left to do but to swallow it, warm down and focus on tomorrow.

After I warmed down and showered, I got back to the hotel around 10pm. I grabbed a bite to eat and turned in for the night. I was completely exhausted from the previous bad night's sleep so collapsed into bed and crashed out. I couldn't believe it when I woke up the next morning at 7am – I hadn't managed a continuous six hours sleep in months. I was feeling much better and pretty positive about the day ahead. I really wanted to do myself justice in the Pursuit. I had been making such good improvements in it in the previous two months I was looking forward to testing myself. I knew at worst I could improve the time I had ridden the 2 km Pursuit in at the Vets Omnium. Not only was I now indoors but I had a super new aero helmet and Aidan Reade had kindly lent me a good pair of wheels – a full Zipp disk for the back and a five spoke for the front. Aidan was a rider from a different club but also the unofficial mechanic and had been helping with everything while I was in Manchester, I don't know what I would have done without him – probably forgotten to pump my wheels or something equally stupid! The wheels were a great bonus to have. Anything that reduces aerodynamic drag is really beneficial in any event on the track but particularly in the Individual Pursuit.

Hugh had written a piece for me to read before the event and I poured over it at breakfast. It went exactly as follows:

"The Pursuit:

We probably have put the biggest body of work into this and improvement was quite dramatic with 14 sec improvement at the Nationals. This was the one which blew me away. Improvement has continued since then as distance came down from 3k to 2k which suits us so much. We have the starts sussed – that 160m and now we are sitting at a higher speed. We have laid down some serious fast laps over recent week and you so have the time of the effort in your head from your efforts on the rollers. We know we can deliver steady watts, know we have the sustained leg speed. We have proved this time and time again on watt bike and rollers. We have worked hard in the windy conditions at Sundrive – well today there is no wind – and a super smooth surface which just wants you to go fast. You have done this so many times in your head and that mental practice will stand to you.

Now you can see what you can do after the extra training, the taper, better equipment and a track that wants you to go fast. You are the perfect build for a pursuiter and your performance in the Nationals is the performance that made everyone sit up and take notice and we have moved on from there. I know you will be happy with how this goes but the real purpose of this is to set a marker from where we push it to the next level. I know you are in the best condition of your life but I also know if you can do all this on the limiting factors that this year brought, then you are capable of so much more.

Go for it! Sustained but steady relaxed power delivered with the cadence that comes from all the practice you have laid down.

This year we have come to understand the attraction of the pursuit and our training methods have kept it enjoyable. We gave only a small proportion of our time to this discipline coming up to the Nationals and yet the gains were huge. Obviously the strength and sprint training we had done helped greatly. We have consolidated that improvement and that base of training is even more suited to a 2k effort. A sprinter who pursuits – their worst nightmare!!

Now well rested – well warmed up and so much specific training done for this.

You are ready!!

This will be like your first dart for the double top!!

Huge belief in all you have done and what you are capable of. I know you see it too. Consistent improvement and all that have been achieved in recent months tells its own story. This is the bonus round – you already have had a kick ass season!!"

As I read this I could feel the belief he had in me coming off the page. And what's more I believed too. Yes of course I was nervous, but I was also quietly confident in a strangely calm way. I was feeling super good this morning, the headache was gone and I was well rested. "It's going to be a good day", I said out loud to myself. After breakfast I headed for the track. The Pursuit heats would be mid-morning and I wanted to make sure I had plenty time down there to chill out and warm up in equal measures properly. For the Individual Pursuit the heats take place in the morning and the top four riders from the heats go into the medal ride-offs that evening – top two ride off for the gold with the loser taking silver, and the third and fourth faster from the heats ride off for the bronze medal. I was just hoping I would get a good draw – the last thing I wanted was to be drawn against someone whom I would catch and have to pass as that would slow me down and diminish my chances of qualifying. I was really hoping all going well I'd manage to scrape into the bronze medal ride off. Looking at the times for last year I'd need to ride about a 2.44 to do this. 2.49 had been my outdoor time and I reckoned I could go five seconds faster indoors so thought it was within my capabilities. However, you can only do your best and whether you make it into the medal ride-offs is completely dependent on who your opponents are on the day. The main reason I wanted to make it into a ride off was that it would double my experience of riding the Pursuit on an indoor track, and lay down a marker for myself for next year.

It seemed, however, it was to be my day. I'm not really a superstitious person but everything just seemed to fall into place and there were signs everywhere. My first stroke of luck was in the draw. I was delighted to see I had been drawn against a British girl, Adel Tyson-Bloor, whom I suspected was a pretty good rider. "Well if she catches me that's her problem", I grinned to myself, thankful that she was good enough that I wouldn't have to face the problem of overtaking her. I was delighted not to be drawn against some of the other girls in my age group whom were even more inexperienced then me at riding indoors and might potentially have a major mishap, like falling off the bike. The other good thing about the draw was as someone who performs well under pressure, I knew that being matched against a good strong rider would force me to lift my game and ride to the best of my capabilities. Therefore who you are matched to ride against in the heats can be very important. Even though the Pursuit is basically an individual time trial, particularly in the qualifying rounds, there is always an element of competition in it. You can just about see your competitor out of the corner of your eye, unless you're catching them of course, but if they are basically level with you it's hard to even get a glimpse of them.

However, everyone will have someone "walking the line" for them, basically a person on your team letting you know if you're up or down on your opponent and by how much or how little. They do this by walking forward or back from the Pursuit start line reflecting how much up or down your opponent is on every lap. They also use hand signals too, which are sometimes hard to understand. I remember in the Nationals as I did my Pursuit wondering as someone was waving their arm up and down at me whether that meant I was ahead or behind! Having someone walking the line for you is important because if you are neck and neck with one lap to go, digging that tiny bit deeper to go a fraction of a second faster can mean the difference between qualifying for a medal ride off and coming fifth.

Comfortable that I had a good draw I set about warming up. Again I had a fixed schedule to follow and relaxed once I was engaged in the process. The warm up for the Pursuit takes about 60 minutes. I was listening to music during my warm up on an iPod borrowed from Hugh, with my large earphones on, their function being to make the statement "don't even talk to me! I'm in the zone" as much as to listen to the music. I found that Florence and the Machine's newest song at the time "Spectrum" had a really good rhythm for the warm up. Whatever it was about the beat it got my legs spinning at the right cadence and helped me visualize riding the laps on the track. It was really upbeat and energizing. I listened to it a few times and as I was winding up the warm up an official came over to me and said – "Susie? It's time to make your way up to the pen". The pen is a square of floor in the center of the velodrome, a central area where the riders ride around slowly waiting to be called to the start gate. I was in the pen for a few minutes when there was an almighty clatter up on the track– two men who were in a Sprint heat came crashing down on top of one another and were lying injured on the trackside. The time ticked on and the word filtered through that one of the guys – a very brave Italian – wanted to have a re-start so they had to scrape him off the ground and have the medics check him over. What this meant for me was I had to kill an extra 15 minutes and try to stay warm. I didn't get too stressed though. I just asked Sean, my Irish teammate to get my rollers so I could keep ticking over. Riding around in the pen is not an effective way of keeping warm. Anyway I stayed calm and things were up and running again pretty quickly. The two other Irish girls in my age group, Geraldine Gill and Ciara Kinch, ended up having to ride off against each other just before me and I was now sitting in the start zone waiting to be called to the gate. Brian Coonan, another Irish competitor, was keeping me company. He had a nice calm way about him and it was keeping me calm. Just as the girls started I suddenly thought I could hear the distant sounds of a tin whistle playing the Irish national anthem. I actually thought I was imagining it first, but after a few notes I said "Am I going mad or can you hear that Brian?!" "Yea, there's some old guy playing the tin whistle – he's been around the last few days playing all sorts of stuff. It's a sign," Brian said smiling. I hoped he was right but regardless it certainly took my mind off the nerves I was feeling. As the Irish girls finished their heat the chunky serious looking female official came over and grabbed my bike. She leaned towards me and said sternly "If you overtake the other rider or they overtake you; you must finish your ride to get a qualifying time. Do you understand?" I nodded and stood up to face the music.

I was pretty amped up by the time the countdown got to the final five beeps and shot out of the gate like a rocket. I had a great start and was absolutely flying for the first two laps when I started to feel it. I realised I had gone out much too fast. I found out after I had just cranked out two ridiculously fast laps so it was no surprise my legs were starting to burn. I was actually starting to see stars by the third lap, and actually had a moment where I thought I was going to pass out. I gathered myself, focused and gritted my teeth, dialing back the pace as much as I dared. Laps four and five I was just hanging by my fingernails as I paid for my over enthusiastic start but I had scrabbled back my effort just in time so was surviving and holding steady. As I rounded the corner and saw three laps to go on the board I thought of something Sean had said to me earlier – "I'm always relieved when I see three on the board – I mean that's less than a minute to go and surely I can push myself and dig deep for that". I also thought back to what I had been reading the previous night. I was in the middle of Gerard Hartman's autobiography and he was describing a meeting with Sean Kelly, one of the greatest Irish cyclists of all time. He had met Sean in the south of France when on a training camp. Apparently Sean had been tested by a sports lab and his physiological parameters such as his VO2 max and lactate threshold had turned out to be pretty average. When the doctors said to him they couldn't understand how he was doing so well with his pretty ordinary physiology he gave them a look and said dryly, in his best Waterford accent I'm sure, "Does that machine measure suffering?" I thought that was brilliant. Gerard had been describing in his book how important things like hard work and an ability to push oneself and to suffer were more important than talent to be a successful athlete. Well as I was in the throes of that last minute I could hear Sean's voice in my head saying those words. "I can suffer too!" I told myself through gritted teeth. With one lap to go I rounded the corner and both my opponents and my bells were rung almost instantaneously. On the track a bell is rung when the riders enters the final lap. Sean roared at me, "You're neck and neck – for God's sake SPRINT!" It was exactly what I needed to hear. My legs had been tying up but I managed to override and keep spinning. I had to dig pretty deep over those last 200 meters as I thought I was dying. I pushed hard and crossed the line and looked up to the board. I couldn't believe my time – 2.38!! What the hell was that? I didn't even dream I was capable of coming close to that figure. I was shocked. I was also momentarily confused looking at the board as Adel's and my times appeared identical. Then I realised not only had I done a savage PB, but I had beaten her by a whisker. I had ridden 3/100's of a second faster than her! Never had I won something by so tight a margin. As I came around to dismount the fatigue hit me in a wave and I collapsed sideways into Sean who had come out to help me off the bike. I was so wasted I couldn't even unclip my feet from the pedals. The reality of what I had done then hit me – I had just ridden a time that would have got me into the gold medal ride off the previous year. "Unless all four of these girls left to ride are amazing I've a good chance of making it into the bronze ride off at least", I thought. I knew I had to get back to my rollers and start spinning out my legs straight away as I had ridden my heart out and would have to do it all again that evening if I was lucky. Within about 10 minutes, however, it became clear as the final pairing finished that I had made it into the gold medal ride-off. I could hardly believe it. I had ridden fast enough that only one girl had gone faster than me. That meant I had won at least a silver medal and I was absolutely ecstatic. I was happy with silver, the pressure was off me now and I didn't care. At that moment I would have taken that silver medal and gone home elated. Gold medal ride off: now that was something! I was on a serious buzz as I warmed down. I rang Hugh and he was so thrilled with me. He said he hoped I'd do a time in the low 2:40's – he couldn't believe how I'd done one better and ridden a 2.38. "That girl you beat is a great rider – she rode a sub four minute 3km indoor Pursuit in the British nationals, I knew she would be tough to beat so well done!" He didn't dwell on this though, and very quickly it was all about focusing on that night. "Now it's all about recovery", he said sternly "get something good to eat and get back to the hotel and chill. Don't talk to anyone except Sean. Get your feet up and lie down for a few hours and make sure you rehydrate". I followed his advice while I was floating. I was still in silver mode. The girl, who I was to ride against that evening, an Australian called Rebecca Wheaton, had ridden two seconds faster than me in qualifying. For me to make up two seconds it was going to be really tough. I talked to Sean about it over lunch. I didn't realise it at the time but Hugh had just spoken to him and sent him off to lunch with me on a mission. "You're going to have to go up a gear", he said to me as we sat down to tuck into our filled baked potatoes. "What", I said "I don't want to! I'll blow up! The last time I did that was for a flying 200m and it made me go slower! It's too risky!" This was my initial reaction. Sean was such a sensible, reasonable guy though he wasn't long in talking me round. "Look", he said. "I saw you. You rode your heart out this morning. You can't go any faster in that gear. You will never go two seconds faster in it and you need to. You have silver in the bag – who cares if you blow up? At least you will have tried." This thinking was further reinforced by Aidan. He assured me, "It's not a big jump. It's only an inch and a half. And with Terry's Mavic wheels you won't even feel it". Terry Cromer, who was one of my club mates from Sundrive, had a pair of top of the range disc wheels, even better than Aidan's, which he was insisting on lending me. I was afraid to borrow them, they were worth so much. He wouldn't hear of it. "You have earned the right to use these wheels. You deserve to have the best chance. You have a real shot at this" he said. "They will make the difference". I couldn't believe the help and support I was getting from everyone. I had about three offers of wheels in the space of an hour. It felt like every Irish person over in the Manchester Velodrome was behind me and wanted me to win. As I was relaxing in my room in the hotel I started thinking about it. The thought had been going around in my head but suddenly confronted me head on. "I have a real shot here at being a World Champion." It was like a revelation. I might never be here again. Even though I was slower by two seconds it seemed everyone around me thought I could do it. I had sent a few texts to friends and it seemed from their replies the people at home were believers as well. After an hour or two in my room I went to meet Sean in the lobby. We had some hot chocolate and he reassured me again that it was the right thing to do to go up a gear. I had completely accepted it at this stage and wasn't worried anymore about it. Rebecca, my opponent for that evening was also staying in the hotel and sitting in the lobby eating a bowl of Weetabix. I watched her for a few minutes. Looked at her demeanor, her body language. All of a sudden the realization just hit me. "I can do this", I thought. "Because I want this more than she does." I knew at that moment how important actually wanting it was and that it might give me the edge I would need.

That evening as I warmed up I listened to the same music again. Every song seemed to have a message for me but a few in particular stood out. Eminem was singing to me "The moment , you own it, you better never let it go, you only get one shot, do not miss your chance to blow, This opportunity comes once in a lifetime". As I listened to Florence singing Spectrum over and over again I couldn't get over the words. It was like this song had also been written for me, the spectrum reflecting the stripes you earn the right to wear as a World Champion. When the official came to bring me to the pen I was ready. Sean and Aidan accompanied me. This time the swarthy official lady had something different to say as she leaned over and grabbed my bike to put it in the gate. "The only difference this time around is that if you catch the other person or get caught the race is over." As she fixed my bike in position she looked at me and smiled with a twinkle in her eye. "Have a good ride!" It seemed like even she was behind me this evening.

After the countdown I started strong and powerful as I had earlier and sat down when I had reached my cruising speed. Again I went out a little hard for the first and second lap, but so had Rebecca so by lap three we were pretty much neck and neck. I settled back the pace a little, this time being determined to keep something for the end. She was slightly up on me but from Sean's reports every lap I knew I was there or thereabouts. I don't think I was ever so focused in a moment in my life before, as I was during the two and half minutes of that gold medal ride. It seemed nothing existed but me and the track, with Sean flashing in and out of my vision every 20 seconds or so. This time I could hardly feel my legs as they spun round. It felt like I was nearly out of my body and watching from above. I even found time to pray and ask God to allow me to get the best out of myself as I went round and round the laps. I don't even remember seeing the lap board. All I remember is the wood, clinging onto the bike, hearing the wind rush past my helmet and the very distant cheers of the crowd, "Come on Susie!", being roared out as I went past the Irish crew. I could also hear one person in particular roaring out my name in an English accent. I found out afterwards it was a steward I had befriended from the previous year at the Masters, David Truman, who was giving it socks roaring for me in the final. I remember registering the lapboard with three laps to go. This is it, less than a minute left, dig deep I breathed. I upped my effort incrementally for these last three laps. I saw a flash of white, yellow and green at the far corner of the track and I realised I must be ever so slightly ahead. As I said before with the Pursuit, you don't actually see your opponent unless you are gaining on them. Sean confirmed that I was up slightly and I kept my focus and put everything into the last two laps. I heard the bells for the final lap ring slightly apart but didn't know who's was rung first so just put my head down, hung on for dear life and dug even deeper as I powered for the line. I hit the finish and there was a moment of silence. It was as if time stopped. I looked at the board for what felt like an age but was really only a second and my name flashed up with a "1" beside it. I let out a massive roar of delight and punched the air. The last ride I had collapsed off my bike in exhaustion, this time I just felt elation and didn't want to stop pedaling. I roared my way around punching the air as I went, "I'm a World Champion!" I shouted, as much at myself as at everyone else. The crowd were loving my excitement and reaction to winning and were cheering and clapping with me as I did my few laps of honor. I finally rolled to a stop into the group of Irish supporters on the side of the track and someone wrapped an Irish flag around me. I got off the bike and simultaneously hugged everyone, then I was surrounded by people jumping around me in delight. I felt so grateful to them all, as all had played a part in the victory, from gear to mechanics to moral support – the importance of having a good team around you for success was never so clear to me as it was at that moment. My one regret was that I wasn't able to cycle for a few laps up on the track with my arms in the air and the flag flying like they do on TV. I decided not to chance it as it would probably end with me in a heap on the ground. I was hardly off the bike when Aidan, my super mechanic, handed me the phone. "Someone wants to talk to you." I knew it had to be Hugh. "I'm a World Champion!" I screamed down the phone at him. He was in shock himself and couldn't take it all in. He congratulated me wholeheartedly and said, "Go off and enjoy this moment now, you can talk to me later when the dust settles." I knew more than anyone he knew what this meant to me, there were no need for words. Everyone was talking at once telling me about what they saw during the ride and how convincingly I had taken her on in the last few laps. I was thrilled when I saw my time, 2.36! I had ridden two whole seconds faster than in the heats, and beaten the Australian by a comfortable half a second in the end. I marveled at the miracle of it all. "The funny thing is Sean, it didn't even feel hard this time, I didn't feel anything at all! It was like a dream. What the hell is all that about?!" I did another celebratory jig with him wrapped in the green white and orange.

After a few minutes as the initial crazy celebrations in the Irish crew were dying down, I was approached by a man called Declan Byrne. He was in charge of anti-doping at the Masters. He was also Irish. "Congratulations, great ride" he started and shook my hand, but he had other fish to fry, "you have to go to anti-doping now. You have half an hour to get yourself ready". "Oh my god I'm being drugs tested", I thought, "I must be good!" I was delighted. I know it sounds strange but it was nearly the icing on the cake for me. It was something I was aspiring to as only elite athletes were drugs tested. I had a chaperone that had to accompany me everywhere for the half hour. "What should I do?" I asked her. She advised me to drink plenty of water so I could produce a sufficient sample. I was all over the place as so much was going on. I rang Cormac to let him know what had happened as soon as I got back across to the warm up zone in the track centre. He actually knew already and was absolutely thrilled for me. He had been following the progress on Facebook, as one of the Irish girls, Sarah Piner, had been putting up live updates on a feed. "Have to go now, I'm being drugs tested", I told him proudly, "call you later!" I then got up on my rollers to try warm down. My head was all over the place though and I actually fell off the bike, landing on top of poor Tonya who was beside me warming up for her event. Thankfully I didn't do her or the bikes any lasting damage. After 20 minutes or so I told my lady friend I was ready and we went down to anti-doping. Sarah accompanied me for a bit of moral support. I was fascinated by the whole process. I managed to just produce the bare minimum, 90 mls for the test so breathed a sigh of relief. It had been kind of hard to pee with the door wide open and a female paramedic standing in the doorway watching my every move! The whole process is very involved and I suppose designed so the athlete being tested can't claim anyone has tampered with their sample. You have to do everything yourself, from selecting a sealed kit of your choice to opening and closing all the tamper proof bottles and pouring your pee into the various containers. There's also a lot of paper work and an opportunity to declare anything you have taken in the last few weeks that might affect your test. "How about beetroot juice?" I asked Declan, eyeballing my jar of pee with its distinctive rose hue, courtesy of those purple veggies. I had been consuming it daily as the latest theory was that it was supposed to improve your aerobic performance, or so Eamonn had informed me. Eamonn was very persuasive, or maybe I was very impressionable but I'd been consuming vast quantities of coconut water (great for hydration and preventing cramp as its full of magnesium) and the beetroot juice ever since he had suggested them a few weeks previous. Declan gave me a bit of a look and jotted it down. "Whatever you want to declare", he answered seriously. Even though I was giddy, this was serious business and he was being very professional. I could see how he would be very good at his job and he would take no attitude. God love anyone facing him who was on something questionable. I'd say he could spot them a mile off.

After all the samples had been collected and paperwork finished I was free to go. When we returned to the main arena nearly an hour later it was almost time for the medals ceremony. Random people were coming up to me and congratulating me and saying things like, "Great ride, really enjoyed watching you". I was delighted. One German guy came up to me and said something I'll never forget, "We need more people to celebrate like you when they win a title. The way you reacted was fantastic! The whole place got to share in your delight at winning. Too many people just roll over the line and don't acknowledge it at all". It was a good point. I had noticed that too. I couldn't understand how people held it in. I went crazy. I suppose it was so unexpected, on so many levels, the victory was all the sweeter and I valued that moment all the more.

The medals ceremony was a big fanfare and I savored every minute of it. The girl who had won bronze in the other ride-off was the British girl I had beaten in my heat. I was delighted she had won a medal as it had been so close between us in the heat. As I lined up in front of the podium with the other girls my eyes welled up with tears. I was so proud. I thought of Tori and wished more than anything she was here so I could hoist her up on the podium with me, as in a strange way she was responsible for me being there. Maybe the pregnancy had had a training effect, and not only that, working around minding her meant I had to train smart. Maybe having her also encouraged me to get out and go training more than I would have as minding a baby can get a bit cabin feverish. Most importantly, however, I think having her had made me mentally tougher and I was able to dig deeper when I needed to. Mental strength was a huge part of being successful as an athlete. I had only learned that this year with the help of my coach. In fact it was just as important as physical condition and training to achieve success.

As we stood there I was first presented with my rainbow jersey and pulled it on with pride, zipping it up to the neck. Then this was followed by the gold UCI medal, and its beautiful rainbow ribbon. We were all presented with flowers and it was time then to stand up on the podium. The podium was huge, so I had to clamber up awkwardly in my cycling shoes. As we stood there and the Irish national anthem played I felt so emotional. A strange desire to laugh and cry all at once filled me. I was as high as a kite. The anthem was impressive, really loud and it reverberated around the track centre. It sounded like there was a full orchestra playing it there at that moment. The flags were raised slowly up to roof level at the far end of the arena with the Irish flag flying high. Then the best bit – they played Chariots of Fire! It's ridiculous but there's something really inspiring about that song and then the tears really did start to flow. I threw my hands up in the air and took it all in. Someone gave me my flag again and I proudly held it up. The two girls hopped up on the rostrum beside me. As I looked up at the flags, it felt great at that moment to be Irish. Representing two nations with a great history of track racing an Aussie on my right and a British girl on my left and an Irish girl had beaten them both. I had wondered how it would feel to be here, as people can have different experiences of winning. Maybe it's to do with your motivations for getting there but some people seem to find it hard to take it all in and it can be an anticlimax and even feel hollow. However as I stood there on one of the best nights of my life, something I had read recently that Fatima Whitbread had said came into my head. When asked about the feeling of standing on the podium after winning the javelin in the 1984 Olympics she replied simply, "If I could take one feeling and bottle it". "I'm with you on this one Fatima", I whispered. I thought she had pretty much had summed it up nicely.

EPILOGUE

When I started writing this book, I had been planning on pulling together all the robust scientific literature available on pregnancy and exercise and basing my advice for women on that. However, I quickly abandoned my initial plan as I realised it was not going to work. There was not going to be any one exercise regime to fit all. I had carried out a survey of exercising mums and I discovered not only is every woman and her ability to tolerate exercise at varying intensities different but every pregnancy is different, and every stage of pregnancy of course is also different. That's a lot of variables to deal with. I If I took this approach I would end up producing a book that was like so many books available already, too vague and over-conservative.

Throughout everything, I kept coming back to the two pieces of advice the Dutch professor gave to me when I wrote to him at the start of my pregnancy. Number one, avoid sports with a high risk of blunt abdominal trauma such as kick-boxing, and number two, listen to your body.

I decided to take up his wise advice and together with all the scientific studies I read during my literature search I came up with a plan for myself. I worked with my coach to devise strategies for safe cycling and to design suitable training plans that I could work on at different stages of my pregnancy. As it happens I was also lucky enough to have a consultant who was very pro-exercise during my pregnancy. I remember one visit when I was 37 weeks pregnant. After he did a quick scan on the baby he asked me what I'd been up to that day and I told him I was just back from an 80km cycle that morning. He didn't bat an eyelid. "Super weather for it", he said. I was glad of his support but I'd long since made up my mind to do my own thing regardless.

That left me with my own recipe for training during my pregnancy, but where did it leave my book? For a few weeks I abandoned the whole idea. As time went on though, I still wanted to write something for other pregnant women out there and I came up with an idea. Instead of telling them what to do, I would tell them what I did, about my experiences and the knowledge I gathered in the process. I would arm them with information to make up their own minds. I knew I had a story to tell, one that was defined by my own personal experiences both during and after pregnancy.

After I had Tori, I realised that there was more to my story than the type of exercise I did in the second trimester. Mine was a story about a woman whose personality was defined by her passion for sport and competition and how she was afraid that pregnancy and becoming a mum might change all that. It was also a story about how she got to grips with coping with becoming a mum and the impact that had on her life. It was during the first few weeks post-partum when I was basically floored that I decided I could help others by telling my story. I knew that when I was feeling a bit low and struggling to cope with this new life I would have loved more than anything to read about someone who was similar to me and also had a bit of a struggle getting to terms with motherhood, and its impact in general. I remember one day when Tori was about three weeks old and having an afternoon nap, I got a chance to sit down, open my laptop and in my sleep deprived state I poured my heart out, which basically turned into Chapter 5 of this book. When I read back on it months later I was glad I had written it down, so much of the hard stuff is forgotten as time goes on. Mother Nature's way of ensuring we go on having more babies I suppose.

The story just kept getting better as the summer went on, with my faster than anticipated return to fitness, the improvements in my cycling and the winning of multiple national medals starting with my first only six weeks post birth. When I started writing I felt it would be good to tell my story spanning a year, ending with the experience at the World Masters in 2012. However, I never dreamed that the story would end with a chapter titled "World Champion". I was so fulfilled after that event I felt that if I never won another thing again in my life I would be happy. The pursuit of a childhood dream to be good at sport was realized and I didn't feel deflated, or wonder "what will I do now?", I was just fulfilled and content. And all of it was done with Tori which added an extra dimension to the success.

I'm now back working two to three days a week as a fish vet, travelling all over the country. It's a new challenge juggling the extra ball of work, along with Tori, my husband and training, but I'm just about managing to keep them all in the air, with the occasional one crashing to the ground on a bad day. Tori is growing fast and every day making new advancements and developing rapidly. It's so much fun to see her change and achieve new things. She never stops moving, just like her mum. Working takes quite a bit out of you physically and mentally and it can definitely be a challenge to find the time and energy to fit exercise in, and more importantly to schedule in some decent rest and recovery time. I try not to miss an opportunity to train even if I'm not 100% up for it. The secret is you just have to try and get the best out of yourself even on the bad days; I know that's what makes a true champion. Having said that I always keep in mind first and foremost training should be fun and enjoyable.

In the latter stage of writing this book I managed to contact and exchange e-mails with Sonia O'Sullivan, the middle distance runner and one of Ireland's most prolific International female athletes ever. I had read her autobiography while in early pregnancy and found it inspiring. There wasn't a huge amount of detail about the exercise she did during pregnancy in the book but the impression I got was she had trained right through and like me, even when she was overdue. Before I mailed her I had always thought that elite athletes would by privy to advice that the rest of us recreational athletes couldn't get. Once we got talking though, it really seemed that she had been in the same boat as me in terms of getting good information and advice about exercising during pregnancy. Sonia had to make a lot of it up herself as she went along, basing what she did on the few facts she could gather and a lot of common sense. She was surprised to hear that things hadn't really improved since she had been in that situation, 10 years previously. When she pointed out that at least now women had the internet to turn to for advice, I told her due to all the misinformation out there it was nearly more of a hindrance then a help. She also had found it so difficult to source information herself, she had contemplated writing a book about her experiences. While she was looking for advice on training during pregnancy she told me she eventually came across a book that had given her the confidence to maintain some sense of normality. I wondered if the book was Dr Clapp's, the one I had found so useful.

After talking to Sonia and a few other athletes who trained through pregnancy, there were a few points that kept coming up. I have made some comments on these aspects that people may find helpful:

Use of heart rate monitors

Most medical people advise that your maximum heart rate (HR) when pregnant should be 140 beats per minute – Sonia remembers she used to laugh at that rule as her HR would be up to 140 going up the stairs at the gym! If you want to use HR, Dr Clapp advises that it is safe to train up to 80% of your max HR, which is a lot more reasonable for most people and will allow them to do a good workout. Or in my opinion just as good an option is chuck out the HR monitor and go on feel - if what you're doing during training doesn't feel strained and difficult; keep on doing it.

Type of exercise during pregnancy

Choose something that works for you and change as required at different stages of pregnancy. If running became uncomfortable, switch to the gym bike, cross trainer or swimming. I found the cross trainer fantastic in later months as you were upright and it alleviated the heartburn I was suffering from. Even if you feel you have to cut down on your chosen sport, don't worry, it's possible to put in the same time and effort into something alternative and maintain your cardiovascular fitness in a different way. It's also a chance to do some cross training or a weights programme, which may even improve your performance in your chosen sport down the line.

Cycling

I cycled about 3,000 km on the road during my pregnancy. I felt that with the rules I had devised with my coach re safe cycling that I was happy enough to be out and about on the road. Nothing is risk free, but there is such a thing as measured risk. I definitely think everyone needs a plan to optimise safety if they are going to continue road cycling during this time. The size of your bump is another consideration – when the bump is small the baby has more protection than if its sticking out and hanging down two feet in front of you. I had intended giving up the bike at 30 weeks but I never got a massive bump so kept going. I loved being on the bike and used to forget I was pregnant. I felt my body had completely adapted to pregnancy near the end and was cycling faster with less effort in the third trimester. Post-partum, my advice is to get back on the bike as soon as you can sit comfortably on the saddle.

Running
If your sport is running, by running regularly each week you won't notice any great changes in your body shape, size or balance. If it starts to become uncomfortable or you get some niggling injuries don't be afraid to let the running go and walk briskly as an alternative or cross train. Only go back running post-partum when your body feels comfortable running again and you are enjoying it. Finally build up distance and the intensity gradually once you start back to avoid injuries.

Gym
I started lifting weights properly only when I became pregnant. I got some advice on good technique which is key to preventing injury. Resistance training is a fantastic way of helping your body not lay down too much fat during pregnancy but is also really good for your moral and self-image. I transformed my bingo wings into a fine pair of toned arms during my pregnancy.
Some gym classes are also suitable. Spinning classes are a way of cycling in a safe environment and you can do them at your own pace (just employ the "fake turn" on the resistance dial!).

Core work
I can't emphasise the importance of core work. Regular sit ups may not be suitable but planks, side planks and core exercises that work your side abs and back are great. Keeping a strong core is crucial for prevention of back pain during pregnancy, and helps one recover strength and shape rapidly post-partum and most importantly it helps prevent injuries when you return to training.

Aerobic boost post-partum
This was something Sonia mentioned to me and I was in total agreement. There are significant improvements in lung capacity, oxygen uptake and VO2max in the few months post-partum and you need to take advantage of these changes when you can, in order to optimise your return to fitness, especially at a high level. Therefor the best time to get out and start training seriously again post baby is basically as soon as you feel up to it post birth. How you feel is a better indicator that the commonly touted "wait 6-weeks" rule. This is an important

time to avoid injury as some of your ligaments may be temporarily lax post pregnancy. Listening to your body is definitely the most important piece of advice to guide you on your return to training.

Surgery and return to exercise post-partum

Like me, many women end up having a caesarean section. This is never usually part of the plan and certainly wasn't part of mine! I was very lucky and recovered very quickly from the surgery. Within three days I was up and about walking around the hospital, within five days going for walks in the neighbourhood and around town. Recommended times to exercising again post-surgery range from about 6-12 weeks. I was back on the track bike within three weeks. I felt that it was the right time for me. Track cycling is generally nice and smooth and you are extremely unlikely to fall off especially when you're not racing so I felt it was a reasonable risk I could take. Approximately 70% of tissue healing post-surgery is completed by 3 weeks, after which point it tapers off. I felt it was a reasonable time to return to exercise for me. I would recommend that it is important to go on feel more than ever here, as some people may be ready to return to exercise as quickly as me, others may need much longer.

Finally, what now of my plans re my cycling? I know I said I don't care if I never won anything again but it turns out I still have the drive for competition. I plan to return to Manchester in 2013 to defend my title and maybe at some stage in the next few years even break the existing world record in my age group. I know it could never feel as special again as it did this time around, but there would be something very nice about being able to call myself multiple-world champion. And who knows what I can do without having to spend most of the intervening year pregnant or in the post-partum phase? I may not even do as well, and I'll know then my success was all a "pregnancy effect". But I plan to give it my all and find out what else I'm capable of. My mother despairs at this and said "I thought you'd give up all that cycling now!" I apologize to her and say maybe next year, just to keep her happy even though I can't see a limit or an end. I suppose it is human nature, to find our limits and strive to push beyond them and that's what makes life worthwhile. That and having babies of course!

November 2013

This is a self-published book and I hope you have enjoyed it.
Follow me on twitter at susie_mitchell or check out my website,
www.pregnancytopodium.com, for updates, pictures and articles.
I would love if you could review my book on Amazon!

9259918R00086

Printed in Great Britain
by Amazon.co.uk, Ltd.,
Marston Gate.